Who Cares?

Supporting my Son through a Mental Illness

Ann J Graham

First Published 2021

Copyright © under exclusive licence to Ann J Graham.

The rights of Ann J Graham have been asserted in accordance with the Copyright, Designs and Patents Act 1998.

No part of this book may be reprinted or reproduced or utilised in any form or by any electronic, mechanical, or other means, now known or hereafter invented, including photocopying and recording, or in any information storage or retrieval system, without permission in writing from Ann J Graham.

ISBN: 978-1-913822-18-7

This book is a inspired by true events. All the major events happened. Some names have been changed to protect the identity of individuals.

'World Mental Health Day is an opportunity for the world to come together and begin redressing the historic neglect of mental health.'

Dr Tedros Adhanom Ghebreyesus, Director-General of the World Health Organization (2020).

Let every day be such an opportunity.

Prologue

The first trip for me was fairly daunting, but it was worth it because I was going to see Paul again. My instructions from the bus company had been to call in two days beforehand to book a seat, which I duly did. The bus would arrive at 8 am at my designated pickup point for the four-hour journey.

That Sunday morning, I was eager. No need for an alarm because I'd been awake for hours before I was due to leave; I could not be late. I had dressed smart but casual and hoped I had it right. Feelings of both happiness and anxiety meant I had checked and double-checked, even triple-checked, all that I intended to take. After all my planning, I opened the door to leave, only to realise I was still wearing my slippers; was this a worrying omen for the day?

It was a typical late autumn Scottish morning when I set off; the streets of the northern city still glistened with what remained of the night's moisture. I put my head down, battling against the bitter breeze and trudged on, reaching the last corner too early for the pickup, but no matter. The streets, including the bus shelter, were deserted.

My usual self-critical thoughts intruded. *Have I got the right day? Have I made a mistake with the time? Have they already gone?*

The panic subsided slightly when, after what seemed a long five minutes, two people sauntered towards me then stopped a few feet away. I could only assume we were waiting for the same free bus down south. We found it hard to avoid eye contact. While I pulled my coat tighter to form a barrier against the early morning air, I surreptitiously observed my travelling companions who were sharing what appeared to be a bar of chocolate. Something told me the elderly man wasn't used to wearing highly polished, brown dress shoes—the giveaway was his blue tracksuit bottoms—but he was obviously used to eating squares of chocolate before 8 am. His equally elderly companion was carrying various bags, one of which was proudly emblazoned with the word *Harrods*.

I thought, *Surely that's not where she bought that silver bomber jacket?*

I hadn't been expecting a luxury coach, so I wasn't surprised to see a minibus arrive with the company name in bright blue standing out against the grubby, grey paintwork. No indication of our destination was showing. Unfamiliar with the procedure, I watched as the driver opened the door.

He shouted, 'Name?' as I left the pavement.

Taking a step up, I gave him my full name and was about to say where I was going when he took his stubby pencil and ticked me off his list. Scanning the queue, again he demanded, 'Name?'

I figured I didn't need to give any more information. One more step and I was on.

The woman with the Harrods bag answered, 'Saint Clair.'

A wry smile flitted across my lips as I thought, *More like chocolate éclair!*

I eased myself up the aisle, with only the briefest of nods traded between me and the few adults already seated. I looked twice at a pair of empty seats midway along the bus, seeking the cleanest, but it was difficult to distinguish the upholstery pattern from the stains. It was a pretty cramped mode of transport and, as I placed my bag on my selected seat, I could see Tracksuit and Bomber Jacket had made it up the bus steps to sit close to the driver.

As we moved off, the tension in the air was tangible, leaving little room for words. Hopeless faces stared ahead, and it didn't seem right even to look around at the others, never mind strike up a conversation. There was no stopping at regular bus stops; we weren't a regular group. Only the driver knew where the next pickup would be: at a road end, beside a park or, for all I knew, a spacecraft terminal.

We headed through the city suburbs then kept going south on the motorway until an hour later we took a detour into a medium-sized town, slowing down as we neared a row of shops. The two waiting passengers were not distinguishable from the general public except that they each stood with full plastic bags and had lost looks on their faces. The response to 'Name?' was 'Kelly'.

Ah, I was learning. Giving the surname was clearly all that was required. Our new arrivals seemed a bit dishevelled.

I silently scolded myself, *Stop this! Stop being so pass-remarkable! Behave yourself!*

However, I came back to my naming game when it soon became clear that something was amiss. Within minutes of us setting off, now complete with the Kellys, a whiff of an unmistakable odour made itself known until, bit by bit, the unpleasant smell filled the bus. Charming. Convinced that someone had opened egg sandwiches, it wasn't much of a challenge to link *smelly* with *Kelly*. I let my head drop, partly in despair and partly to bury it in my book after reminding myself that we were all in the same boat, so to speak.

Two hours into our journey that first Sunday, the driver made his last pickup. After the Kellys, I had refused to more than glance at any additional boarding passengers for fear of losing it completely. The driver closed the door for the last time and, apart from the engine roar or the indicator rhythm, only a selection of softly spoken words penetrated the silence.

We must have been ten minutes into the last leg of our journey when a loud, shrill female voice startled me.

'It's not his teeth!'

I looked up from my book, wondering if I'd see someone holding a pair of lost dentures. A muffled mumble came from the male sitting next to Shrill Voice. If you can have an argumentative mumble, then that's what it was.

Shrill Voice countered this. 'I'm telling you, it's them tablets. They make him disentorientated.'

I had to question myself. *Did she just say that? Is that even a word?*

With a final muffled mumble, I concluded that the man had lost the argument; it was the tablets that were to blame and not the teeth.

I so wanted to be off that bus.

From then on, I allowed the remaining two hours of the journey to become an opportunity to contemplate the good and bad that life had thrown at me and my family. I could not help but let my thoughts drift between visions of the baby, the boy, the teenager and now the young man who had, irrevocably, changed his own life.

As the sun surrendered to the invading clouds, rain threatened to fall. Trying to put my thoughts into perspective and plan for the future, I was scarcely aware when we passed through hamlets and villages where women hung out washing, children played with dogs and men cleaned cars. Now and again, the traffic built up and the few shops that traded on Sundays opened their doors. No one paid attention to the dozen downcast travellers passing by in an insignificant vehicle.

We interrupted our trip with a 45-minute comfort break at an indoor shopping centre. This was an opportunity that nobody wanted to miss; for me, it was a fleeting chance to mix with normal people who were spending the day buying new clothes or window shopping, having coffees in cafés or strolling with families. We couldn't be normal people that day; we were committed to less normal endeavours.

Our break over, we were counted back onto the bus. I had scarcely resumed my seat when the grey clouds overhead darkened the already bleak atmosphere inside the bus. Raindrops ran down the window like a torrent of tears, attempting to expose my fragile mood to the world.

Things became seriously tense and quiet much later when, after driving out of one small town, the road narrowed and the countryside opened up. The landscape displayed a few forlorn farms, a playful pony and a well-worn tractor. The sense of calm outside stood in contrast to the unrest within me.

Gradually, the views changed and I could see what I figured was our destination in the distance. The long, tarred road skirting the fields appeared alien in a setting where a trodden pathway would have seemed more natural. A solitary blackbird, finding its balance on a broken fence, bowed its head in reverence to our now deathly silent group. We were approaching what looked like an abandoned building surrounded by sprawling fields devoid of trees, animals or farm buildings. High fences greeted us as our driver stopped in his allocated parking place, leaving room for other anxious visitors.

We had arrived.

BOOK ONE

Chapter 1

A Young Life

The meaning of Paul is the Little One and, as a little one, Paul was a contented baby. He was quick to sleep through the night and rarely cried. I had recently divorced so, as a very young, single mother, circumstances dictated that I was responsible for providing newborn Paul and his four-year-old sister, Cait, with safety, love and support to build their way in the world. Compared to those many mothers with difficult children, I was lucky.

By the time he was approaching two, I could see in him the contrast between complete contentment and extreme emotions. He was a cheerful boy, but he often broke his heart if he couldn't master something quickly or when things were not going well; he felt the disappointment more keenly than others around him. One problem I encountered early on was when I tried to teach Paul how to feed himself; the whole frustrating procedure devastated him. He couldn't quite get his coordination going and the food reached the floor faster than he could get it into his mouth. Calmness resumed when he eventually learned how to master the basics of finding his mouth rather than his right ear. I appreciated he could well be the type of boy who felt the intensity and pain of frustration until he was eventually coaxed through to tranquility.

As a toddler, he loved the times spent at playgroups and crèches, he couldn't wait to fling his jacket off and get started. He would look in amazement at the other crying children whose mothers were trying hard to convince them it would be fun inside. They would point to Paul to encourage their little ones. 'Look at that boy. He's going to play with all the toys. Why don't you go in now?'

Paul wasn't afraid to leave his comfort zone in the secure knowledge that I'd be back for him. This early realisation would provide a coping mechanism for him much later in his life.

His special toys were usually action figures who wore a uniform. While watching his favourite TV programmes, it was important for him to get into character. He would dress up in red underpants over black footless tights to convert himself into Superman; he truly believed the tea towel pinned around his neck gave him that authentic look. When we moved to a new house, he had his own Action Man-themed bedroom; however, he struggled to keep his room in some semblance of order. He could never find anything. Socks and pants went missing but there was one constant – the place where the red underpants and leggings were kept, always on hand for the Superman transformation.

Once he reached school age, he expressed a desire to join groups like cubs, sea cadets and even a karate club. The problem was that he wanted the uniform before he joined, and even when I explained that most boys go for a few weeks to see if they really like the group, he would have none of it. He would try once but never go back. The uniform was important to him because, in his mind, somehow it denoted stability and belonging. It wasn't difficult to detect that, like any youngster, Paul wanted to be a *big boy* but only if that came with approval.

'Mum, please can I say bad words?' piped up four-year-old Paul one day with a curious expression on his face.

I wondered what was coming next. I responded in a calm voice, 'Oh, that's an interesting question. Which words would you like to say?'

At that, he rhymed off a few coarse swear words.

I replied, 'Hmm, well we could think about it. Do you know anyone who says these words?'

'Yes, some of the boys outside.'

After a moment I continued, 'You know that boy, Kevin, who lives in the white house? I've heard him saying bad words, and I don't like him very much.'

I could see him pondering this before I heard, 'I don't think I'll bother saying bad words.'

He especially valued praise from his teachers; however, school itself was never going to be a favourite place for Paul. Socialising by rolling down the mudslide near the playground was one thing but having to go into class and learn was not so appealing. Teachers complained that he was slow compared with the others; calling me in to listen to examples of star readers and look at the maths tests results of the top students while I tried to figure out a way to interest Paul in what he thought was a complete waste of time. That was unless something interesting was taking place in class. A pirate ship project was one such event.

The children were asked to bring in something to construct and enhance Pirates' Corner. They could provide accessories, hats or swords, anything that pirates might wear or use. We had nothing I could think of until Paul found a rope in the garden shed; a huge, heavy and extremely dirty rope that had been used to tow cars. After much discussion, when he had insisted it would be perfect to cordon off Pirates' Corner, I gave in and helped him to school with the dreaded rope concealed in a large plastic bag. When he arrived home later that day, he was beaming, announcing proudly that the teacher had praised him for his idea.

The next day, he came home with his school report. He sat grinning, waiting in anticipation of what praise his teacher would give him. I read it out, but quickly the smile dropped from his face. She had written, *Paul needs to stop capering in class.* Gutted, he was out to get revenge. At the end of school the following day, I looked out to see him dragging the unravelling rope along the pavement and onto the garden path. He abandoned it by the rose bushes and threw his bag down.

In a bitter voice, he announced, 'She's not getting the rope. She put rotten things about me in that paper.'

I asked him what he'd said to the teacher.

He replied, 'I just said, "My mum wants her rope back!"'

He didn't get what he wanted, so he pulled out completely and, as he saw it, got his revenge. I could imagine him furiously extracting the rope from the display.

He began to struggle to come to grips with the real world, especially if exacting revenge for what he considered unfair acts was outside his control. Despite a certain amount of innocence, there was a cunning side to Paul. He was beginning to understand what he needed to do to keep his head above water. He was very good at making up a story to sidestep something he didn't like or was struggling with. Nowadays, teachers are quicker to detect children who can't keep up and help can be offered. Paul might have had a different experience if such facilities had been available in his primary education.

One day, I had been running errands after taking delivery of a bathroom shower cabinet. Paul arrived home from school at his usual time.

'Where have you been, Mum?' he scolded. 'My teacher has been trying to call you for ages because I've been ill.'

He told me he'd had a really sore stomach, but as far as I could see, he looked fine. As soon as he saw the shower cabinet, his eyes opened wide; he abandoned his schoolbag and rushed towards it.

'Yeah! A Doctor Who box!' he exclaimed.

The mysterious stomach ache had disappeared and while he was jumping in and out of the shower cabinet, he announced he was hungry. Sitting with him as he munched his way through a sandwich, I asked what the class had been doing before he became ill.

'Learning to tell the time,' he replied.

It didn't surprise me he'd become ill. Paul could not grasp the hours and minutes of the analogue clock and I realised he'd cleverly feigned illness for practically a whole school day. The irony was, of course, he'd fallen behind even further and had to face the same topic later in the week. He wouldn't have got away with another illness. At parents' night, I told his astounded teacher of his ploy; his performance had fooled her. We tried, unsuccessfully, to master telling the time together until I had to give in and hire a maths tutor to help. Paul had discovered avoidance tactics that could be used to his benefit.

Yet, he also had a passion for testing himself to the limit. 'Look what I can do!' He followed this with a request for me to count the seconds while he stood on his head or held his breath underwater. A favourite was for me to tickle his feet while he focused on something else and didn't laugh. Just like any other youngster, he was proud to push himself and extend his limits.

One year, he wrote his letter to Santa Claus asking for a bike. I played down the bike scenario, telling him I believed Santa was struggling that year with big toys. As it was, I had bought him a second-hand, black, BMX bike. On Christmas morning when he opened the living room door and saw the bike, he gasped. Almost in tears, he said, 'You're the best mum in the world!'

I realised from his reaction that he knew it wasn't Santa who was providing the presents. I said nothing more about Santa and I guessed he was too scared to broach the subject for fear of not getting Christmas presents in the future. It surprised me he had kept the knowledge of a non-existent Santa to himself.

Although we had had the odd mother and son run-in, Paul was basically a good boy who wanted to do well and was an obedient child. But I won't play down the difficulties of being a single mother – it wasn't easy. The only respite I had was when one or other of the children was being cared for elsewhere, and that only happened when Paul was staying overnight with his father. Then I could breathe a little; I could meet a friend, read a book or even watch TV without distraction. At times like these, I saw the benefit of having more than one person care for a child. Sadly, Paul never had two full-time parents. He was desperate to see his father, but Cait was more interested in staying with her friends. Our informal arrangement meant the door was open for her to visit him; however, although only a teenager, she questioned his demeanour and attitude towards women. Increasingly, she heard him slighting and badmouthing females; me in particular. She preferred to avoid his company and let him and Paul enjoy *boys' talk*.

On the odd occasion, Paul got into mischief and I smacked him. Corporal punishment was not only permitted then but also encouraged – the adage was: s*pare the rod and spoil the child.* The idea behind this saying was that if a child did something wrong, they had to be punished, and with a rod or stick if possible, otherwise they would never learn and consequently become spoiled. A smack didn't happen very often, but when it did, it left me feeling extremely guilty. I thought, *What am I doing to this child?*

Any compassion was smothered by my irritation and anger at being a single mother. Looking back, it has become clear to me that I didn't want to smack *Paul*. I wanted to smack *his father* for not being there.

However, as much as I could, I had provided Paul and Cait with a full and active childhood in which they were regularly in touch with aunts and uncles, cousins and grandparents. Maybe the treasure hunts and well-hidden gifts at birthdays and Christmases simply weren't enough for Paul and, similar to other children, he wanted more.

The innocence, contentment and happiness that permeated his early years began to crumble when he realised he couldn't be a superhero or fool the teachers. I had done my best, but he was becoming attracted to a different life with his father, a hundred miles away.

Chapter 2

A New Life

Paul normally spent his school holidays at his father's house in central Scotland. Although he had bonded with classmates in his local school, he also built up friendships with the boys where his father lived and felt as though he belonged there too. The pull was not so much the friends, but his father. He had a car; he had money, and he didn't make Paul tidy his bedroom or go to school. That world beckoned him so much that, perhaps inevitably, he pleaded with me to let him live there permanently when he was about to enter his last year of primary school. My doubting instincts took over as I felt things wouldn't go well if he left home.

However, whatever Paul thought of me, he had his father on a pedestal. He loved being able to go to a bar with him, play a game of pool and have a Coca-Cola. In the garage, their talk about cars and dismantling machinery was right up his street. On more than one occasion, when he couldn't join his father, I had to watch Paul break his heart. He would sob, 'Why can't I go with Dad? Why has he left me? He's going somewhere where you can get Coca-Cola and he's not taking me.'

It was more than just being with his father; it was his father's lifestyle and an environment that Paul perceived to be attractive. If I bought him Coca-Cola in a cafe, it would never match the same experience in his father's company and the chance to be a step away from becoming *a man*.

In my consideration, at eleven years old, he was too young to make such a life-changing decision. But, after trying to encourage him to stay with me, I realised he had set his heart – his tears and begging proved that.

There was a condition attached to Paul's departure; it could only happen if his paternal grandmother would agree to look after him while his father was working. I had asked Paul's father if his parents agreed to this arrangement but he seemed surprised that he would have been expected to ask them. He assumed he would have built-in childminders. I asked him to make sure they knew what they were taking on so that neither they nor Paul would be disappointed.

Reluctantly, at the start of the six-week summer holiday break, I helped Paul pack a suitcase and a holdall. His name was put down on the new school roll for his final year in primary. Part of me was sad to see him go but I was also happy for him because I genuinely hoped with all my heart that the move to live with his father would fulfil his needs. Had I persevered, perhaps forcing him to stay with me, he could have fought me all the way, then, when he was sixteen and of legal age to go, he may have left anyway. I knew I'd miss him, but I wondered if it was maybe time for Paul to see the world through the eyes of a male figure in his life.

The house was suddenly different; quiet and tidy. Accepting the situation, the next day I busied myself cleaning his room, preparing it for the school holiday in October when he would come back to visit us. With new, coloured storage boxes for the scattering of toys he'd left behind, and the bedding and curtains washed and ironed, his room looked welcoming but for some unknown reason, I had left an ironing board leaning against the wall.

As suspected, and with a heavy heart, I watched my worst fears slowly becoming a reality as things inevitably began to crumble for Paul. Only 48 hours after his departure, I got a call to say he would have to come back more or less immediately. Staying long-term turned out to be impossible. In fact, even staying for the remainder of the summer was to be cut short. His father's work schedule changed and travel plans were imminent. Paul's grandfather was angry that he hadn't been consulted about what he saw as an eleven-year-old being dumped on him and his wife. He demanded that Paul be sent back to me where he belonged.

I was pleased that Paul still had his friends nearby and arranged that he would be able to join his old primary class again when school started; after all, he'd only been away for a few weeks of the summer break. At the back of my mind, however, I wondered if I'd have a battle on my hands. I hoped we'd be a united family again and I'd be able to watch him grow into a young man. Unfortunately, Paul was not happy at all with the arrangement and, once home, quickly demonstrated his fury. I was the cat he thought he could kick. He was angry and frustrated because, as he saw it, his world was caving in. The day he arrived back, he hung about the living room and sat staring into space for a short while. He half-heartedly joined in the conversation. Once we had returned his clothes and toys to his bedroom I passed a comment about keeping some of his books and puzzles tidy in the new boxes so he could easily find them.

To my astonishment, he slowly looked me up and down, behaviour I'd experienced before from his father but never expected from eleven-year-old Paul. Then with a snarl on his lips, he spat out, 'Tidy? In here?' He made a sweeping gesture with his arm in the direction of the ironing board and continued, 'Tidy? Half the things in here aren't even mine!'

This was the sarcasm I had seen in his father and didn't like. I could tell bad habits were forming. Between the derogatory look and belittling comment, my first instinct was to retaliate. Reacting in the moment, I verbally struck back.

I asked him to sit on the bed as I explained, 'You're right, Paul. Half the things in here aren't yours. In fact, nothing in this room is yours. I paid for it so it's all mine: the wardrobe, the bed, the desk. Also, your clothes are mine. I paid for them too, but I'm going to let you keep wearing them. I'm going to let you keep using all the things in this house that I've paid for, so you don't need to worry. And you can stay here as long as you want. We want you here, but we don't want bad manners.'

There was no need to say anymore. I felt he was beginning to go in the wrong direction as far as his attitude towards me was concerned, and perhaps indeed towards other females. However, I eventually realised that, despite my harsh response, a more respectful young boy began to emerge over the next few months.

Normal life resumed. Paul rekindled old friendships and went into his final year at primary school but even though he continued to stay with his father during the holidays, he still longed for a solution that would allow him to live there permanently. He seldom picked up his old toys and the

Action Man bedroom that had been his pride and joy now paled into insignificance. I knew he was growing up and would be expecting less boyish surroundings, but my limited budget couldn't manage a room makeover at that time – another nail in my coffin.

Circumstances changed a year down the line. His paternal grandmother had been widowed and Paul was delighted to hear that she and his father had joined forces. They had moved into a bigger house, which would allow Paul to live there with them. He had the choice of how his new bedroom would be decorated and he would have two adults to support him through his teenage years. So Paul, now twelve years old, left home and school for good during these summer holidays; he was ready to start term one of his first year at secondary school. As had been previously agreed, some roles would be reversed and now he would come back to me during most of the school holidays if possible.

That July day, Paul was demonstrably over the moon, moving out for the last time. I watched him through the window as he ran back and forward, filling up his father's car. He had packed a few things the day before, but now he was making last-minute decisions about what to take. His heart must have been beating like crazy, spilling over with happiness and excitement; unlike mine. I felt my body deflate, moving from emptiness to complete abandonment over a very simple and innocent thing.

He picked up a picture and, taking care to walk rather than run this time, gently placed it in the already packed boot of the car. It was a silver-framed photograph of Paul proudly kneeling beside a friend's dog with our typical Scottish scene of hills surrounding a loch in the background.

I thought, *He's even taking the picture!*

I said nothing to spoil his fun, but he wanted to remove all traces of himself from me. I was to be an extra; distanced from him. I felt a certain amount of guilt that I hadn't been able to provide what he wanted in his life. Deep down, I knew his grandmother would provide for him, but I was worried that the woman who had brought up his father was now going to bring up my son. My concern centred on her being an older woman with values that gave the male figures in her life inflated importance. Paul's father had run rings around her, and my intuition told me she would allow Paul to do the same, possibly devaluing a woman's worth in his eyes.

Over the following weeks and months, I realised I now had no major responsibilities. Cait was sixteen years old and attending school in a nearby city. An outgoing girl, she had made friends from far and wide and was becoming more and more independent. We spoke about Paul and looked forward to planning family time when he visited. As a typical sixteen-year-old, Cait was involved with school and growing up. Although she said she missed her brother, the days, weeks and months went by so quickly that it seemed no time until he was paying us another visit. Her life was full and we all kept in touch by phone and letter. I must admit that not only was I pleased that someone else would be responsible for Paul, but also I felt this was an opportunity for me, with space of my own, to do something worthwhile. I didn't have to be home at school closing times and the absence of extra washing, cooking and tidying up meant I had time on my hands. I wanted to make the best use of that precious commodity and fill the void, so I decided to get myself an education and enrolled at a local college.

Soon after Paul left, his best friend Will from primary school came to visit me. All he wanted to do was to sit and talk about Paul; he was missing him too. When I mentioned that Paul would be coming back to visit in a few months, Will promised to visit again. So, in December, Paul arrived and waited a few days to see if Will would turn up. When he didn't, Paul set off in search of his pal. He remembered the street Will lived in but not the door number. As he approached a row of houses he thought might be the right one, in the distance he could see a much taller Will closing a garden gate and walking away in the opposite direction. He hadn't seen Paul, who had also stretched quite a bit.

Paul hollered, 'Will, Will!'

Will turned around but, not recognising Paul, ran in the opposite direction as if a starting pistol had gone off. Paul came home disappointed and bewildered by Will's reaction because he was setting off for his father's the following day and had missed the opportunity to catch up with an old friend.

He tried to make light of it. 'You should have seen him run, Mum. He must have thought I was someone else. Maybe he's done something and figured I was out to beat him up. If you'd seen the height of him, it should have been me running away!'

There were no mobile phones or social media then to track people and so, sadly, Paul lost the connections he had made as a young boy.

The period of Paul's life when he lived with his father was a fragmented time for me as I watched him grow up from a distance. I didn't get to see very many copies of school reports so, apart from what Paul told me, I never really knew what was going on regarding his subject levels, attendance or behaviour at school. I knew he enjoyed craft and design (woodwork) in his third year at secondary school and, on one visit back home, he puffed up as he handed me a spice rack he'd finished making in class. He had fashioned it in such a way that it was supposed to hold six small spice jars, so I transferred my spice jars into it one at a time. When I got to number five, it was clear there wasn't enough space for number six; he physically deflated when he saw his mistake, but I reassured him.

'No, no, that's fine,' I told him. 'It's much better if there's only five in it because then I can get my fingers around each jar, which makes it easier to pull them out.'

We were both content.

When he was about to leave to go back to his father's, he sat, nodding his head. 'Mum, you are the only one who appreciates what I make – everyone else points out my mistakes.'

It took little to encourage him and make him feel he'd done a good job, but it left me with the feeling that he was struggling to be appreciated in his chosen new life.

His early teenage years passed and, as his father often worked away from home, his grandmother continued to look after him. It was a trying time for both young and old. I visited when I could and I saw he wasn't being much of a help to her. All I could do was to remind him that, just as he liked praise and help, his grandmother would appreciate that too. That advice seemed to fall on deaf ears.

Regrettably, Paul got himself into a bit of bother. I came to hear that one night, along with some younger lads, he and his friends broke into a garage. The idea wasn't to steal anything, only to have somewhere to sit out of the biting Scottish weather to have the proverbial cigarette; this was their attempt at being *grown up*. They were caught. At sixteen, Paul was the oldest and so, while the others got off with a warning, the police could charge him. I hadn't been told anything of this incident at the time; it must have been stressful for his grandmother to deal with, particularly as his father was working away. Because Paul had to appear in front of a juvenile court with an adult, his grandmother had to step in. They gave him a year's probation, during which time he would be in serious trouble if he offended again; the next step would have been an approved school.

When I found out, I was deeply disappointed because I thought he had respect for the law. I was not going to be the disillusioned mother who laid the blame at the door of the others in the group; he was sixteen and of legal age to work, marry and have his own children. Perish the thought. Society deemed him to be an adult and, like many sixteen-year-olds in my opinion, he was a long way from taking on such responsibilities.

Now and again, I got the feeling that Paul missed his old life with us; indications that he was divided filtered through. During a short school holiday, Paul brought a friend, Callum, to stay with me. During the day they went out and about, getting up to what boys of that age do. In the evenings, between family and friends who gathered in the house, there was lots of hilarity and banter back and forth. It was good to watch as I could see Paul was turning into a nice young man with a wicked sense of humour. As they were leaving to get the bus back down south, Callum went out first when suddenly, at the front door, Paul about turned.

'I need to wash my hands,' he muttered as he brushed past me.

I was puzzled, but only for an instant before I realised what was going on. I followed him into the bathroom where we hugged goodbye. It probably wouldn't have been cool to be seen hugging your mum in front of your pal. It was a lovely gesture.

I thought, *He's still my Paul.*

A few days after the boys had left, I discussed with Cait how I thought he was getting on at school and how happy he seemed with his decision.

She stopped what she was doing and looked directly at me. 'Mum,' she protested, 'what you don't realise is that Paul knows he's made a big mistake.'

I was stunned. I'd always thought that during the time he had been away from us he was settled and enjoying life with his father. This needed to be addressed. However, he was, in my mind, at a crucial time in school, now in fourth year, and didn't need any more disruption. Sadly, it was years later when Paul finally disclosed to me how much he had been bullied in secondary school. Therefore, with the lack of any further insight into his 'big mistake', I decided to leave well alone. One thing was certain – Paul was never prevented from going to stay with his father or from coming back to stay with me.

However, somewhere in the back of his mind, he must have felt that he couldn't have the best of both worlds without an emotional fight. Once during a school holiday with me, he came out with a random comment. Shaking his head slightly at me, he announced in a firm voice, 'My dad will never stop me from seeing my mum,' but before I could respond, he continued, 'and my mum will never stop me from seeing my dad.'

I agreed with him, but he quickly changed the subject and I was left wondering if he, or someone else, had caused him to doubt his security with those who purported to love him.

When he had first talked about moving to his father's house, I considered his opinions and his voice had been heard, unlike a generation before when a simple request for a new pencil, never mind a request to leave home, would have been met with derision. The *children should be seen and not heard* days were gone. There was never a notion of him having made his bed and having to lie in it, as had been the experience of many. Once, having left home, young people in years gone by would have found their bedrooms changed into a spare room, or at worst, rented out to some stranger. Even though I was sure that as a typical teenager, Paul would have pushed the limits with me but, had he decided to come home, he would have been made welcome. I made certain on his subsequent visits he could speak to me directly about his choice. However, he never picked up on the chance and it wasn't long before he had made a life-changing decision that wasn't to include any family.

I was pleased when I heard some of the things Paul was doing with his life. He was attracted to the Army Cadets and, as I had suspected, he was passing through the unsettled teenage years. Unlike previous attempts at being part of a group, he stuck with his choice and finally had a uniform. He felt as though he belonged. Outside the cadets, the usual teenage events were unfolding. Girls were phoning to ask him out on dates and vice versa; he was a popular lad with a network of friends. Although we wrote and had the occasional phone call, I felt I was missing out on some very important and formative years with him as his visits back to me understandably became less and less.

Six years had passed with Paul being in and out of my life. However, his life in the Army Cadets went from strength to strength, so much so that shortly before his 18th birthday, after he finished school, he signed up for the British Army. A whole new world of opportunities was opening up for him.

As he left home again to become a soldier in May 1992, I had to ask myself, *How can this be? What has become of the little boy I remember?*

With his rucksack packed, he headed off to start his basic training in the south of England, five hundred miles away from everyone he knew in Scotland. I guess I was the same as most mothers who watch their children spread their wings; a mixture of pride and apprehension. I would have been happier to see him develop his practical skills and work nearer home, but the main thing was that he was happy. I remembered witnessing some of his first successes while I stood proudly in the background. When he mastered riding a bike without me running at his side holding the seat or when he finally remembered his lines in the school show as he glimpsed me from the stage in the front row. But I cringed as I thought about the swimming lesson where I had peeked through a window to watch his first attempt at submerging himself. I had had to turn away as I saw him being practically dragged screaming into the water by the instructor.

I hoped for the best but wondered if he would survive in the army.

Chapter 3

Joining Up

Regrettably, I couldn't attend Paul's passing-out parade in Woolwich, England, when he officially became part of the British Army. The final day at Woolwich had been special to Paul, as it would be for any young man, and I had tried everything I could think of to get there, but professional obligations prevented me. Since studying at college, my career had taken me in a direction I had never dreamed possible and, at that time, I was heavily involved with a new job. His father had given us a few days' notice and, in such a short time, it proved impossible to organise travel arrangements, even supposing I could have deferred my work appointments. Unfortunately, Cait couldn't attend either as she was studying abroad. It was some consolation to know his father was there at Woolwich on Paul's transition from recruit to fully fledged soldier. It seemed to me that my two children were now happy with their chosen pathways in life.

I was delighted when I received photographs of Paul's special day in September 1992. I admit to having a tear in my eye when I saw the tall, handsome, young man. The pure white of his belt, epaulettes and gloved hands in sharp contrast to the dark green of his dress uniform made an impressive image. With his thumbs in the *standing to attention* position and his regimental badge meticulously centred on the red band of his hat, he proudly beamed out to the camera. I had wanted to be there.

Eventually, he gave me some stories about those early days in Woolwich. He'd been apprehensive about moving so far away from everyone; in fact, the first day he arrived for his basic training was one he wouldn't easily forget. Several young men joined at the same time and so that first night would have been a prime opportunity to get to know one another. Recruits, in sections of six, were each assigned a bunk in a room within their barracks. They tentatively gathered in their sections and introduced themselves. Paul watched as they filtered away and he waited for his name to come up. After the last six names were called, there was a bit of confusion. Paul found himself standing alone. It seemed there was one person too many for the ten rooms; Paul realised that, unfortunately, due to a clerical error he was number sixty-one. As he would soon discover in the army, there was never an explanation; no reassurance that things would be OK or that he didn't need to worry.

'Follow me!' was the order barked out and, like a lost sheep, he was shown into another barracks, an empty barracks!

Apart from neatly made-up bunks, the artificial light was the only thing that filled the eerie silence. He was told to choose any bunk he liked; he wouldn't have company. Whilst the others would no doubt be chatting, laughing and getting to know one another, Paul was alone. He spent most of the night wondering if he'd done the right thing in joining up. However, the following day everything was sorted. He joined a section and his training began in earnest.

Something that always stuck in my mind was that, right from the start, Paul was encouraged to develop a mindset where he didn't have a family at home anymore. To create unity and a sense of duty between the soldiers, they were expected to switch loyalties, pulling away from the tug of those they'd left behind to connect with their fellow soldiers. In fact, the purpose of the section of six was to have a small number of recruits bond early on. They were kept in their sections for various tasks and exercises and expected to have each other's backs. Leaders and followers eventually emerged; the section essentially took on the role of the family.

The notion that he might be allowed visits during his three-month basic training wasn't spoken about, we knew that he would have a strict regime to follow. As we understood it, there was no real chance of a reprieve except for a forty-eight-hour leave within the first eight weeks and, if possible, a visit from a relative. With no immediate family in the area, Paul wasn't expecting anything other than to stay put with others who were distanced from family and friends. Given the miles between Woolwich and the north of Scotland, we all accepted the situation.

However, as chance would have it, Woolwich was about an hour's drive from Kent where my parents, Paul's maternal grandparents, were holidaying during this period. Unbeknown to him, one Sunday they decided to make their way over to the barracks. His grandfather was familiar with the ways of life in the army and knew that, without an appointment, they could but try to see him. Arriving at the gates, his grandfather, full of pride, told the gate guard that his grandson was in camp. He explained that they were down from Scotland on holiday and would only be in the area for a few hours. He asked what the chances were of being able to see Paul and take him out for a short while. The officer told him to wait while he made a phone call. Returning to the car, his grandfather announced to his grandmother, 'OK, it looks like he's going to sort it out but I'm going to tell you something. You have to remember, Paul is a soldier now. If and when he comes out you can't be giving him cuddles and suchlike. He's a man – he's in the army now – he can't be seen to be cuddling you.'

'Oh, I think he'll want a cuddle from his grandmother,' came the reply.

Minutes later, they saw Paul running like the wind towards the base gate, although not in army uniform, certainly appearing to be obeying orders. He didn't look over to their car but kept his gaze fixed firmly towards the gatehouse. Paul stopped abruptly and stood to attention. As they spoke, the gate guard pointed to the car. Paul turned to look, screwed up his eyes in disbelief, picked up the pace and darted out of the gate towards the car. The first thing he did was wrap his arms around his grandmother, giving her a big hug. His grandmother looked over at his grandfather. She smiled and said proudly, 'See, I told you!'

Then Paul shook hands, like a man, with his grandfather. His grandparents found it amusing when Paul told them he had been sitting in the mess when his training corporal had come in and pointed at him. He hollered an order at Paul, 'Get your civvy kit on and get to the gate. You've got a two-hour pass to spend with your grandparents.'

Paul had jumped up but replied that there must be some mistake – his grandparents lived in Scotland and this request couldn't be for him.

Again, the order came. 'Get over there. Now!'

He was about to repeat his concern about the mix-up, but the training corporal turned on his heel and left. Paul knew he had no option but to obey the order; he pulled a jumper over his T-shirt and ran as fast as he could to clear up the misunderstanding. He was flabbergasted and speechless when he saw his grandparents waving furiously at him. Only the elderly could have got away with that. They spent an enjoyable afternoon together and the short time out became a special memory for them all.

Once the new recruits were ready to leave Woolwich, they were given a list of what the army expected of them and they quickly found out how important it was for them to stay focused. At eighteen years of age, Paul would soon head off on deployment to Hohne, Germany, to join the Royal Artillery, excited about what the future held for him. I wondered why he was going to Germany until I realised that, although there had been a programme of withdrawal of British Forces since the fall of the Berlin Wall in 1989, the army still maintained a presence and sent young soldiers there directly after their basic training in the UK. When we spoke on the phone after Paul's passing-out parade, we promised to meet up on his next leave, even if it meant me travelling to central Scotland, his home for over six years.

Predictably, Paul's chosen career wasn't a bed of roses. He had to come to grips with hard work and a disciplined approach to all aspects of living. On many occasions, he told me I did not know what went on in the army and, of course, he was right. On leave, he would describe incidents, mainly minor ones, that went on within his regiment whilst in Germany.

He recounted some practical joking between the lads in the early days in Hohne. On occasion, they had to go on training exercises, using maps and following compass directions over extremely challenging terrain. On one exercise, they had to gather at a particular rendezvous point; by the time Paul arrived, the others had already started their rations. Famished, Paul took a bite from his sandwich but was momentarily distracted as another soldier dropped something. He laid his sandwich down to help. Then, after he had picked it up and taken another couple of bites, the others burst out laughing. Puzzled, he asked what was so funny.

They screamed with laughter. 'You've just eaten rabbit shit!'

Naturally, he reeled back and looked in horror at the sandwich.

One of them chuckled and piped up, 'No, no. We're only joking. You're all right. Carry on!'

As he explained, whether or not it was true, he found it impossible to eat any more. So he went hungry and had to continue with the second half of the exercise to the point of collapse.

He couldn't report something like this without consequences. It had been a prank; he would have been mocked by his superiors and perhaps punished by the others if he'd even tried to complain. As he remembered this story, his demeanour changed from animated to flat as, no doubt, he visualised the scene and perhaps similar goings-on. The details of the story alerted me to something perhaps not being quite right. Previously I wouldn't have been surprised to have heard that it was Paul who had instigated the practical joke; instead, the experience disturbed him. In his youth, Paul had been a trusting soul and to a certain extent, he still was. The practical joking in the army made him grow up quickly; he was surrounded by young men who were up for a prank at the expense of others and if he couldn't beat them, he'd have to join them.

Another incident happened one workday when Paul and another soldier had been given a task inside the camp, moving equipment from one area to another. It was a tiresome manual job. Paul admitted that they thought it was a ridiculous undertaking as they knew the following day it would all be moved back again. He said that after an hour or so of labouring in the heat, they decided to take a break. As I understood it, they would not have been allowed to rest until they were given a specific order to stop. However, as they stood thinking about what to do next, Paul's version of the story was that an officer passed by and questioned them about the job. This officer also suggested it was a fruitless exercise and, according to Paul, said that the job was no longer required. Apparently, he dismissed them with verbal permission to leave camp. I later found out that, even if the story had been true, Paul would have known he should never have left the camp without written permission.

Off they went and had a superb time on a sunny summer's day, only to face the music on their return. No one would listen to their story, believing that they had taken it upon themselves to have a self-administered break. Surprisingly, or maybe not, neither of them knew the officer who had dismissed them and so it was only their word that was available. They were given a joint rollicking before punishment was meted out. They were ordered by the corporal to stand, dressed in uniform, with a backpack on for hours in the heat. When they were on the verge of collapse, the corporal asked Paul if he wanted to throw in the towel before the time was up.

He drew himself up with determination. 'No, Sir!' came the resounding reply.

Paul said he would never forget the feeling of being sure his legs were going to buckle while the sweat ran down his face and body. Whether they had taken it upon themselves to pull a fast one, or if there really had been an officer who had given them verbal authorisation, that was the last time he left camp without written permission. Fortunately for both of them, this was treated as a minor breach. He could have been told he was forfeiting a month's pay, which would have hit him where it hurt most.

Sadly, Paul's paternal grandmother passed away when he was still in Germany. His father didn't pass on the news until she had been buried and this weighed heavily on Paul. He couldn't understand why he hadn't been told earlier, and by the time he got the news, it was too late to apply for leave to go home. He would have been given compassionate leave that wouldn't have been taken off his holiday entitlement and he definitely would have been allowed to grieve with the support of family. As it was, he was on his own with his thoughts while army life carried on; the minutiae of the day-to-day chores didn't permit him to mourn the female figure who had been instrumental in rearing him during his teenage years. This was an unresolved cruel blow in the background while other episodes occurred.

I learned that once, while on exercise, his section of six was canoeing in rapids. It all sounded very exciting and no doubt the young lads would be daring and over-adventurous as they weaved their way around boulders and rocks, in and out of the deep or shallow parts of the river. They worked as a team and were expected to keep an eye on one another. At one point, they had been told to roll over in their canoes and become completely submerged. Their task was to hold their breath until they could right themselves or escape without assistance. Most of them managed to pop their heads up to a round of applause. Afterwards, one of the group told Paul, when it came to his turn, he rolled over while the others watched for him to reappear. They waited but he never emerged. They glanced at each other and then at their group leader, then back to the overturned canoe. No Paul. On the command of their leader, two of them jumped in and scrambled underneath to release him. When he eventually made it to the shore, he seemed slightly shaken but otherwise fine. No one knew what had happened. He didn't need any medical attention but, for me at least, I wasn't sure if this was a story that highlighted simply his disorientation, a blackout or an attempt to put his own life in danger. Or was it merely a throwback to when he was younger and wanted to be the one who could hold his breath the longest underwater?

There was, of course, time for socialising in camp, when soldiers would meet up in small groups. They tried to make up activities that were riskier than the last to relieve some of the tension; typical behaviour of bored young men together. One night, once all the jokes and hilarity had been exhausted, one of them produced a gun, an illegal trophy of war, and they agreed to play Russian roulette. They were using a very rare and antique gun where most of the chambers had been taped off. Sitting around a table, one of them spun the gun and it ended up pointing between two of them, and after some light banter back and forth, they spun it again. Eventually, it stopped, this time pointing directly at Paul. The group went silent as he surveyed the gun for what must have seemed a second too long.

Before anyone could say anything, Paul shrugged his shoulders and said, 'Oh well, I guess this one's for me.'

He picked up the gun, put his finger on the trigger and pointed it at his temple. He later recalled with a smirk on his face, 'Mum, you've never seen a room clear so quickly! They all jumped up, knocking over chairs as they scrambled for the door.'

On one hand, I guess that could have been construed as a joke between the lads, but I got the feeling that the rest of the group thought there could have been a strong possibility of Paul firing the gun. Their punishment would have far exceeded standing in the sun with a backpack. Military police would have become involved; the soldiers would have been court-martialled, likely charged with attempted murder, with serious consequences.

I wasn't aware of all the goings-on in Germany, but, apart from the few laddish things on the surface, Paul seemed settled. I didn't detect any major problems when he had leave and I enjoyed his letters and phone calls.

During one phone call in August 1994, he told me he was being posted to Bosnia the following month.

'Bosnia? Why are you going to Bosnia?'

'Mum, don't you watch the news? There's a war on there,' he scolded.

I joked, 'I know, but why are you going? You can't even manage to keep your bedroom tidy! What use will you be over there?'

He took it in good spirits. I didn't know what he would have to contend with or what role he would play. I could tell from his voice he was excited. I had to be in the moment with him, but underneath I was fighting against the impulse to dwell on what I had heard about the Troubles in Northern Ireland and trusted that he wouldn't be put in similar danger in Bosnia.

Chapter 4

Theatre of War

Once I appreciated what was going on in Bosnia, I could only wonder how Paul would remain unscathed by what he was about to witness. After his experiences there, he was able to speak about worrying instances where he witnessed maltreatment of soldiers and civilians alike. He told of times when he was sure he was breaking down with the burden of guilt because he couldn't be of help and also of times when he had feared for his life. These experiences scarred him much more than the pranks and jokes in Germany.

Finding himself in a war zone, army life took on a whole new perspective for Paul. The Bosnian War had raged since 1992. Most of the local Bosnian Muslims had been expelled from Bosnia and Herzegovina, victims of ethnic cleansing. The United Nations Forces had refused to intervene in the war, but two years after it started, UN Protection Force (UNPROFOR) troops provided humanitarian aid to the innocent civilians trying to survive in a war-torn country. This was the umbrella under which Paul was deployed to Bosnia between 1994 and 1996.

While there, Paul played several roles, from Basic Radar Operator and Basic Signaller to Assistant Physical Training

Instructor (APTI). He told me that, on his first tour of Bosnia and armed with a weapon, for a time he felt a sense of control on guard duty at the entrance to the base. As in any country where there are young soldiers, the locals are prone to show an interest, especially curious children. The town had been badly affected by the war, resulting in many people having to live on very little, begging and often sleeping on the streets. The poor, hungry children were mesmerised by what was going on with the soldiers. The young ones would often try to speak to the guards in broken English and use their hands in some kind of sign language. It sounded as though guard duty was a relatively relaxed affair; the soldiers didn't stand to attention unless an officer passed, and most of their time was spent sitting on or leaning against a wall. They didn't expect any trouble at the base and so the children were allowed to stay in the area, playing and talking to the guards; I guess more than one blind eye was turned.

Some local Bosnian children were regulars, wondering if the soldiers could find them any trainers or cigarettes. Paul deduced that, even if the children didn't want the things for themselves, they would have sold them on or exchanged them for food. A girl of around thirteen seemed to be the ringleader of one small group. Although she was poorly dressed, she held herself proudly, oozing confidence. With long hair curling down her back, she carried herself like a much older teenager. She often appeared with her younger brother and three or four others of about ten years old, all ragamuffin-type kids.

At one point, when these children were having a bit of fun with the guards, an unmarked vehicle drew up and two burly men got out. As he was telling me, I could see by a shift in

Paul's body language that something disturbing was about to be revealed. He gripped the arms of the chair and his voice wavered as he tried to control his anxiety. He said that the men spoke to the girl for a minute in their native language before bundling her, like an old blanket, into the back seat. Wearing a uniform of sorts, it seems they briefly looked at the guards, mouthed a word that could have been interpreted as *police* and made it known they were taking the girl away. Paul said neither he nor the other guard had any idea who these men were. The confusion between Bosnian Muslims, Serbs, Croats, military and police was exacerbated when some victims became perpetrators and vice versa; things changed daily. Outside their own commanding officers, the soldiers didn't know who had authority. Paul remembered how he felt as the men drove off. He was at a loss as to what he should do; in fact, there was nothing he could do. As he watched them leave, the girl turned round to look out of the back window, eyes wide with fear. Here was Paul, armed with a weapon, witnessing what he believed to be some sort of abduction but unable to do anything to prevent it. His job was to guard the entrance to the camp, nothing more. He was powerless to stop the men and, although they could have been local police, he wasn't convinced that was the case.

About an hour and a half later, the vehicle returned and the sniggering men threw the unsteady girl back out onto the street. As they drove away, once again Paul was left feeling completely helpless. He could see from her dishevelled appearance, the redness around her eyes and the scratches on her arms that more than likely she had been abused in some way by at least the two unknown men. Now here she was, discarded. He had no option but to leave well alone. He and the other guard had been in a hopeless situation and he reminded me that the soldiers continually felt despair at this type of treatment, towards both boys and girls.

His experience didn't end there. Paul was a fish out of water as he witnessed similar incidents when he was sent on a second tour of Bosnia in November 1994. He saw many more distressing situations and was unable to put them behind him. He said his head swirled with negative thoughts. Day and night, he was a tormented soul, and every defence mechanism in his body had told him to get out, but that was impossible.

He insisted that things often appeared unfair, as would be expected in war. Some soldiers were given more difficult tasks than others and didn't feel they had recourse to complain. After all, that was the job they'd signed up for. However, he recounted situations where the lives of some of his colleagues were put in extreme danger after being given what they considered to be unnecessary tasks by their commanding officer. As he relived the scenes, he interjected with rhetorical questions.

'Can you believe he made us crawl through that field knowing that there could be mines or other traps?'

'Do you think anyone would believe he forced us to drive trucks through forbidden streets where a massacre had taken place days before?'

'What commanding officer would tell you NOT to help the screaming children who were clinging to our jackets? We were told to get into our trucks and leave; the mothers were pleading with us to take their kids to safety.'

'We were supposed to be peace-keeping, but they ordered us to leave the men and young boys who were being dragged away by the scruff of their necks or at gunpoint. Why could we not at least try to break things up? I mean, *we* had weapons as well.'

He said he had wanted to ask for some help with his mental state in Bosnia, but the only person he could talk to was the chaplain. He knew in his heart he needed a more qualified person, so he abandoned that idea. He also thought maybe he would bounce back after some rest and recuperation (R&R) in Split with the others, so he waited until his second tour was over and he was back in Germany to analyse what he was feeling internally. He wondered if talking would reveal a weakness that didn't sit well with the image of a soldier. And so, amid the Bosnian War, he fought his own battle, one he felt he was losing.

When he heard that fellow soldiers had been shot at by snipers or mortally wounded in other incidents, it convinced him he was on the verge of a mental breakdown. He ended up counting the hours and minutes until he would be out of there. He didn't know where his next deployment would be, but he was sure he had seen enough of war-torn Bosnia with two tours now under his belt.

He welcomed leave back home in Scotland and in this more peaceful environment, he tried to rationalise what he was feeling. Paul had brought Sam, a pleasant young Englishman, with him. They enjoyed each other's company and appeared relatively relaxed as they spoke about their dreams for the future. Both young men had different ideas about where they wanted their army careers to go. Paul had enjoyed his role as an APTI while Sam's dream was to link up with the Royal Signals; motorbikes were his passion. With his application well on the way to being accepted, he had only another few weeks left before he could join. Sam had had different army experiences – and so he displayed a relatively peaceful demeanour, but Paul was tormented repeatedly as he had flashbacks to abductions and shootings. As these thoughts dominated, Paul told me he wondered if his mind was slowly becoming removed from reality and, more than ever, felt he would make enquiries about support when he was back with his regiment.

He knew the army was his profession and he wouldn't be able to shy away from his responsibilities; not that he wanted to complain, but he instinctively felt something was amiss. He returned to Germany, but nothing had changed mentally for Paul. He was finding it difficult to cope. He couldn't eat and he couldn't sleep. Tentatively, he asked the others how he could go about talking to someone. Before he found out the procedure regarding doctors or counsellors, the worst was yet to come.

He became deeply troubled when he was told he had a third tour of Bosnia coming up in January 1996. The time he had spent in Scotland seemed a million years away as now he kept visualising what lay ahead. He knew as a soldier he had seen things that ordinary people wouldn't be able to imagine, and his thoughts flitted back and forth between his last two tours. With no doubt in his mind, Paul knew he would not cope well with a third tour. He again felt trapped by the intricacies of the profession he had chosen and knew that he'd have to go through the correct official channels to get their expert advice.

He asked around and found out that the doctor was the person to approach. He would try to explain as best he could that he could not face Bosnia again. He put it off for a few days. Feeling as though he couldn't maintain emotional control, he spoke to the doctor. The appointment did not go well, and he felt the doctor wasn't listening. Paul had no choice but to walk away, with no further discussion.

Shortly afterwards, and feeling brave enough to talk again, he made another appointment. This time he asked the doctor if he could speak with perhaps the army psychiatrist or psychologist. He was told that it wasn't possible because the person in question was skiing. As he voiced the word 'skiing' to me, there was more than a hint of scorn in his voice. Here he was, a soldier who had looked death in the eye and was falling apart; now he was being told the only person who might be able to help him was having fun. He walked away from the doctor again. I got the impression he had been so confused at this point he didn't know where to turn.

As a last resort, one avenue that might have been open was approaching his superiors directly. He could lay it on the line and ask for their expert opinion. He certainly was given advice but he didn't expect it to take the turn it did.

When Paul finally told his superiors he was struggling, he was pleased to be told they'd find a way to deal with it. He was called back a few days later to be informed that they had a replacement for him on the tour. Momentarily, Paul breathed a sigh of relief. Then he was informed that Sam, his fellow soldier and the very friend who had been to Scotland with him, could go in his place. That was such a shock to Paul – he knew both of their worlds would collapse because of this decision, and it seemed to him that his superiors knew this as well. Paul was devastated, as was Sam, but the decision was final. As a result, with a posting to Bosnia pending, Sam's request to join the motorcycle team was put on hold and, into the bargain and by way of a final blow, Paul was told that the army had reconsidered and he would now be joining Sam and the others in Bosnia anyway. This kind of treatment was all about obeying orders and clearly he wasn't. He was told, as all soldiers were, that's what he was being paid for and so they responded to his objection by giving him a short, sharp shock. Both young men were dumbstruck, with Paul feeling overwhelming guilt that he had likely cost his friend his lifelong dream. His problems hadn't been resolved, they had escalated.

Paul couldn't tell me how he felt as he had prepared for Bosnia for the third time. He had no words to describe his emotions. Along with the others, the two young men knew they faced many traumas and upsetting scenes; it was part and parcel of their life now, so they had to try hard to control their angst.

One distressing memory Paul was able to speak about from this third tour was when he and Sam were in charge of driving an army truck to a destination several miles away. The soldiers were instructed never to go through the town, where the crowd would jeer and attacks on vehicles weren't uncommon. Not everyone in Bosnia wanted foreign military intervention. When they had covered most of their journey, they found themselves on a deserted, extremely rough, country road where they spied a roadblock in the distance. It was difficult for them to tell how many vehicles were there and who might be manning this blockade, be it official or otherwise. They decided that, although it was risky, the best idea would be to turn around and try to find a different route. A decision had to be made, and through the town it was. Sam was driving and soon realised they were heading into a populated area, putting themselves in jeopardy. With rising anxiety, they agreed to get through the forbidden route as quickly as possible.

The roads in town weren't busy with vehicles but there were people on the pavements and others crossing roads. The pedestrians soon caught sight of the army truck and began staring and pointing. They were driving past a group of people when, out of the corner of his eye, Paul saw a man step off the pavement in the direction of the side of the truck. They felt a distinct thud and the truck rattled. They glanced wide-eyed at each other. In unison, they choked, 'Keep driving!'

Realising they would probably be lynched if they stepped out to see what had happened, they never even looked back. They consoled themselves by thinking they might have run over a rock on the road or that something had been thrown at the truck. Voicing the words to me later, Paul reminded himself that they had both feared the worst scenario. What if they had run into someone? As this part of the story unfolded, his voice was controlled but the fear in his eyes betrayed his inner torment. In his mind, they could have run over someone and he was, once again, racked with debilitating guilt.

However, their troubles were not quite over yet. Before they were completely through town, their unease heightened as they faced yet another roadblock that forced them down what was known as Sniper's Alley, so-called because they would be within range of the snipers' guns trained on passers-by. The tension was unbearable and their adrenaline peaked. They froze when a single shot rang out. They knew they couldn't stop as they would be immediately gunned down or surrounded by locals; even if they didn't stop they could still be ambushed if they drove too slowly. Again their voices rang out, 'Keep going!'

Having driven out of town, they were able to relax a bit. When they were sure they weren't being followed, and in a state of emotional turmoil, they burst out laughing; gallows humour. Neither of them thought the situation was remotely funny, their rushing adrenaline had made it all too much.

Once safely inside the base and pretty shook up, they sat for a minute as they thought about what to do next. They turned to each other and Sam said, 'Well, are we going to look?'

They held their breath as they circled the truck. At the right-hand rear side, there was a mass of indistinguishable, pale pink matter partway up, which had further splattered as they had continued driving. For sure they would be in trouble, first of all for going through the town and secondly for potentially being involved in an accident without reporting it. They couldn't ignore it so, running the risk of punishment, they told their superior the full story.

His response was, 'Wash it!'

Although there were no repercussions at the time, Paul was to be haunted by the incident for years. He spent many an anxious day or night believing that they might have killed someone in the street and that, as a consequence, the family would track him down to punish and torture him. They never discovered the truth of the matter. Ultimately, the uncertainty of what took place made him fear the worst, and the guilt that he felt for perhaps taking a life was agonising.

A ceasefire ended the fighting in 1995 after a massacre in Srebrenica, when around 7,000 Muslim men and boys were murdered and 20,000 civilians were expelled under yet another ethnic cleansing process. All this left deep emotional scars on surviving soldiers who had tried their best to bring aid and protection through UNPROFOR. For Paul, the stress of three tours in Bosnia never completely evaporated.

Chapter 5

Time to Leave

Following each of his three 12-week tours in Bosnia, Paul had to return to base in Germany. On the face of it, everything seemed to be going well for him there – he had a steady income, a bunch of friends and it wasn't long before he had a lovely girlfriend, Dee. Trips outside the camp became an attractive reward for hard work; meeting up with friends, chatting over a coffee or a beer were most welcome opportunities for relaxation. Paul was impressed by the German system and the cleanliness of the country, with its stringent rules for recycling and controlling pollution. He had no problem with the strictness of the German authorities and never questioned their laws. It seemed, at that time, the army had taught him respect for authority, rules and regulations.

He also kept his promise and came back to visit Scotland when he could. There were times when I would drive to the Central Belt to see him on leave; sometimes he would come to me. Now and again he was on his own but, more often than not, he brought a fellow soldier to meet the family. Not surprisingly, he eventually preferred to spend his time off in Germany. He was part of a small group of soldiers who seemed to stick together through thick and thin, although they were at different stages of their army careers. He was spending time travelling during his R&R, exploring Germany and taking the occasional trip to Holland. The time finally came when Paul wanted to take advantage of the opportunity to live in off-base accommodation where Dee could join him. He was still gainfully employed in the army and was obliged to turn up for work every day; she worked in a café/restaurant near their flat.

He built up a group of friends, a few of whom were not attached to the army, and this whetted his appetite for more freedom. He was mastering the German language, albeit from friends, and so he could communicate and mix with the locals in his free time. Although he had some pleasant experiences, now and again when he was on leave, I sensed tension and mistrust of others in him. It didn't come as a complete surprise when, soon after his last tour of Bosnia in April 1996, Paul gave the standard six months' notice to his superiors. With three tours of Bosnia and training exercises in Canada and Poland behind him, four years and one hundred and fifty-three days of army life ended.

During his last six months, he was approached on more than one occasion by his superiors who tried to encourage him to stay, but he felt burned out and knew it was time to leave. He needed a change; he didn't know what kind of life he wanted, but he knew that he didn't want any more of the army. When I learned this, his decision rang alarm bells. This hadn't been the first time Paul had walked away from a secure environment without concrete plans. I reflected on the boy who had left home at twelve and grown into the young man who left home again aged eighteen to join the forces. The army conditioned him to become an extremely tidy man, one who was often capable of quietly thinking out what his next steps would be. Now, at twenty-two, he had finished serving his country and he was, yet again, ready to move on.

This time he had a different mindset which, perhaps because of his experiences in war-torn Bosnia, didn't always appear to be stable; he wasn't quite the same person who had joined up four years earlier. Despite his positive plans for a future with Dee, I detected a change in his mental health.

To a certain extent, I was encouraged by the stability he had managed to find outside of the immediate family. However, I was disappointed to hear that his departure from army life wasn't dealt with in the most sensible way. He intended to stay in Germany and had plans to rent private accommodation. He loved Germany and didn't want anything to scupper his chances of the happy life he was planning. Somewhere in his unsettled mind, he had thoughts that the army might put obstacles in his way. To combat this, he wasn't entirely truthful when army officials asked what his intentions were following his discharge. He lied to them, saying he was going home to Scotland. Army provision ended there as he was supposedly going back to the support of his family.

I suppose I secretly hoped that he would settle down and focus on learning a trade. His interest in mechanics and how things worked might have taken him in a direction where he could have trained as a car mechanic or in some type of engineering. Although maybe older than others who embarked on such a career, he would have had good reason for his late start. I had wanted to speak to him about getting a qualification in the UK that would stand him in good stead for any other country, including the Germany he loved. However, there was a cloud hanging over this idea. Paul didn't always want to go through the nitty-gritty of learning from the start; he preferred to jump in a couple of levels higher without knowing or appreciating that achievement comes from building up from the basics.

Taking a step back, I had to remember that I didn't know the real Paul. I hadn't been around during his secondary schooling and I wasn't convinced I knew all of the ups and downs associated with his adolescence. I never witnessed his interactions with friends and, although I had been delighted that he stuck with the cadets, I didn't know if it had all been plain sailing.

At that time, it seemed he knew the German system and would more than likely have contacts there for housing and work. From that point of view, if he had settled in Germany, as a family we would have had the opportunity to visit him and see life from a different perspective. It struck me that he might not have too much of a problem making Germany his permanent home because, as a boy of twelve, he had made the move to his father's house and, as I thought at the time, hadn't fallen apart.

Initially, all Paul wanted was a steady income and a nice life with Dee. He didn't have concrete plans for his future and was prepared to take things one day at a time. However, after only a matter of months of leaving army life, a pattern began to emerge; when he became emotionally unsettled, he became physically unsettled. Consequently, he flitted between Germany and the UK, finding neither peace of mind nor stability in either. In both countries, jobs and relationships suffered. He never had much money; his tentative plans for the future weren't coming to fruition and he seemed to go from one mishap to the other.

The stories that straddled the two years after he left the army were a clear indication that, in Germany, without the necessary paperwork or knowledge of how the system worked, he was in a bad place. Despite coming from a profession where he had become adept at driving an army truck, keeping physically fit and handling a weapon, he was finding that these skills weren't called for by many companies. As a result, the only way he could survive in Civvy Street was to take temporary, part-time, low-paid posts such as being a security doorman or helping in transport yards. Into the bargain, he often had to contend with being the last to be hired and the first to be laid off. He struggled to take orders from new bosses; they didn't wield the same power that his army superiors had. These jobs gave him money in his hand, but not the security needed to survive everyday life.

Although Dee and Paul lived together, they could barely afford even a low rent. As was normal between their groups of friends, everyone chipped in and helped with bits and pieces of furniture or kitchen goods to get them off to a good start. Paul brought Dee to Scotland on holiday and I was a very proud mum when I initially saw them together. This was the first time I had seen my son in a serious relationship and I hoped he'd found something special with this lovely person. With her long blonde hair and off-the-shoulder baseball jacket over her petite frame, she was the epitome of what I realised was his dream girl. He had always liked the Kylie Minogue lookalikes and Dee was practically her double. She seemed head over heels for Paul but I was disappointed to learn that he often appeared socially awkward, was more than a little selfish and, most worrisome, was demonstrating signs of paranoia.

During their time with me, when Dee and I had some time alone, I was sometimes surprised to see him appear out of nowhere; that was typical behaviour he would have seen in his father. As she and I sat in the garden, Paul would miraculously materialise from around the corner when we thought he was indoors. If we found ourselves casually chatting on the sofa, after a few minutes he would pop his head around the door and ask her to come with him for a moment. I didn't see anything wrong with a young man wanting to be with his girlfriend all the time, but it was her reaction that bothered me. The happy, relaxed, chatty girl suddenly became compliant and with her head bowed she would follow him; this made me wonder if he was bullying or abusing her, again learned behaviour.

I couldn't help but probe a bit further because, in her, I recognised my own unhappy self from many years previously. I learned from Dee that Paul very seldom offered to help out around the house and what she told me about his condescending remarks to her made me realise his attitude towards females was definitely questionable. I had suspected this might be the case all those years before when he challenged me about the ironing board in his bedroom. Dee reluctantly told me she felt manipulated regarding the clothes she wore and he questioned her every move. In my opinion, he appeared insecure and controlling. But I had to wonder if there was some throwback to the trauma of his army experiences, which hadn't helped his mental health and was now affecting their relationship.

Much later, when he came to visit alone, I was to hear of a strange and alarming story about when they were driving to a friend's house. They stopped at a garage so that Dee could buy cigarettes. Paul had stayed in the car and when she came out he told her that, although he was parked a distance away and the car radio was switched off, he could hear what she and the man behind the counter were saying through the radio waves.

He said to me, 'And can you believe it, Mum? She looked surprised that I could hear everything they had said. Then she put her head in her hands and asked me to take her back home.'

When we discussed it later on, that hadn't been the first time he'd either heard voices or instructions through the radio or television. On and off, he'd been telling Dee about the voices and in the end, recognised that she was scared although he couldn't understand why.

She was loyal and caring, but he was spoiling what they had together. He was scared she would leave him, but his actions were pushing her in the very direction he was trying to steer her away from and, finally, they split up. Neither of them knew how to cope. Their parting of the ways could be put down to two young people finding it difficult to adjust to life together, but there's no doubt his questionable mental state worried her. Eventually, it came to light that this was nothing compared to some other characteristics that were manifesting themselves but sadly were left untreated.

It wasn't all about voices; his very perception of life didn't always seem to be rational then. Years down the line, he told me of an incident after he had split up with Dee and was still living in Germany. Friends had invited him to a party on the other side of town but he didn't have a car, so it took him half an hour to travel there by bus. He was one of the first to arrive and, as people started joining the party, he realised he knew most of them. However, during the evening, he glanced around and spied a man he didn't know. Paul had a good look at what the man was wearing, and his shoes caught Paul's attention. Paul had the same type of shoes at home, the same colour with the same design at the front, and in fact, the leather at the front of the man's shoes had creased in the same places as it had on Paul's shoes. By now he was staring at the shoes and convinced himself that the man was wearing the shoes that should be in Paul's cupboard at home. He couldn't figure it out. Automatically, I wanted to suggest that they had both bought the same shoes. However, this intrigued me and I wanted to figure out how Paul's mind was working, so I asked what he thought had happened.

'Well, before the party started, he must have found out where I lived, waited until I'd left, then gone into the flat and taken my shoes from the cupboard.' He stated this as if it should be clear to anyone. He told me he didn't want to say anything at the time because then he would alert the man to the fact that he had caught him out.

I probed further. 'So how would he have been able to get into your flat?'

He glanced at me, expressionless. 'Look, Mum, what you don't realise is how easy it is to get into these flats. Anyone who knows what they're doing can slip in a small, hard card, like a credit card, right where the lock is and then it's simple.'

The farfetched possibility that a stranger would watch Paul's comings and goings to break into his flat to take a pair of worn shoes failed to convince me. I really expected Paul to burst out laughing and say something like, 'Got you there, eh?' However, something about his demeanour was telling me that even at the moment of our conversation, he still firmly believed his version of events. I couldn't dismiss his story because I wanted to hear how on earth it would end.

Hoping he wouldn't clam up, I asked, 'So how could you categorically tell that the man was wearing your shoes?'

'Simple,' he snorted. 'I've told you, the creases were in the same places as on my shoes. I just had to double-check by looking in my cupboard.'

He continued, saying he had left the party telling no one, got the bus home and ran up the stairs to his flat as quickly as possible. The lock on the door didn't appear damaged and so he took hold of the handle through his tee shirt to make sure he didn't disturb any fingerprints. Once inside, he tentatively opened the cupboard door and… there were his brogue shoes. He told me the man had put the shoes back in the cupboard in exactly the same place. I asked him what he thought had happened, and he explained that the man must have had a car, realised the game was up at the party and got across town quicker than Paul. He'd left the shoes in the cupboard, thinking that Paul wouldn't be able to prove he'd taken them. With such an incredible story, he appeared to be unravelling. His circle of friends was steadily decreasing and such a distorted perception of reality likely caused friction with even his closest allies.

Chapter 6

Worrying Times

Trying to lead a normal life was becoming a strain. If there was no job, there was no money, and the German benefits system had been difficult for Paul to navigate. He received weekly payments in arrears, and he was often paying his benefit to those he had borrowed from the week before. At one point, Paul lived in a block of flats near a few friends. One young lady and her mother, who were concerned for Paul, would invite him to visit at mealtimes. He revealed to the mother that things weren't going well for him and he was worried because he couldn't keep control of his finances. I suspect she had previously advised her own family and so tried her best to help Paul. She asked him to bring a note of all his incomings and outgoings and kindly drew up a plan for him that showed that he wasn't at rock bottom as he'd thought. Although this was a sympathetic gesture, it left Paul thinking he didn't need to change his lifestyle. If there were any suggestions about tightening his belt, he didn't disclose them to me. Even though he barely had enough to make ends meet, he had continued to mismanage his money without considering the consequences. Now and again, other friends would step in and support him with a bit of cash here and there, but that was a big ask. Most of them were in the same situation, having left the army at more or less the same time as Paul. Life was tough enough between trying to build up relationships and survive outside the protection of the army, where food and a bed had been readily available. Paul continued to have mounting debts and eventually couldn't afford his own place, so he took to sharing or sofa-surfing. He told me he eventually realised he had to get a grip on his impoverished existence.

Once he found that surviving in Germany without the support of the army wasn't quite as easy as he'd thought, he came back to Scotland. But the same patterns of being emotionally and physically unsettled were mirrored in the UK. Life had not always been a bed of roses in Scotland. A few incidents during his teenage years had created tension between him and his father. However, Paul still had contact with friends who welcomed him. A good friend, Steve, had been in the army before Paul and knew something of what he was going through. Steve had parents, brothers and sisters to support him and, unlike many ex-soldiers who don't make it in Civvy Street, he had been able to hold it together and make a life for himself. I hear of many homeless and mentally ill men who have at one time served in the army and it is only through good fortune and some lasting friendships that Paul and Steve avoided being cast aside by society.

Although Paul had a period of socialising with old buddies, there was no sign of any real employment, which meant he wouldn't be paying his way and, naturally, this eventually caused a rift between him and some others.

As far as I knew, he wasn't making much of his life in Scotland but it still came as a surprise when one day I got a phone call from his father to say that he was about to have Paul arrested. His version of the story was that in a bar, Paul had asked his father to buy him a drink. His father refused and an altercation broke out. Paul left, went back to the house where they were living, found a crowbar and proceeded to smash the windows of the family car. Knowing there would be a price to pay, he quickly grabbed a few belongings and left.

I'd like to have known more of the story, but it was clear that the conflict and animosity between him and his father had finally reached a breaking point. The police were informed but it took them some time to eventually locate Paul. He was arrested and charged. Yet another run-in with the police. As an offending adult, he was ordered to appear a few weeks down the line at the local Sheriff's Court. He called me to explain. When I found out what was happening, I asked if he'd been able to talk to someone about the situation. He gave me the name of his court-appointed solicitor. I was permitted to contact him and, although I knew Paul was in trouble, I wanted to know more and maybe explain that I suspected an underlying mental health issue. I wasn't trying to have any sentence or fine reduced, I was trying to find out how I could prevent such a situation from arising again. I called the solicitor and he told me he had visited Paul as soon as he had been arrested but Paul wouldn't talk to him.

'It was like trying to get blood from a stone. He wouldn't tell me much about his background or give a straight answer to my questions,' he quite openly told me.

I explained. 'I am sure you told him exactly who you were, but I'm not convinced Paul would have understood your position nor would he realise you were there to help him. He would have seen you as a figure connected to the court system and probably thought anything he told you would be twisted and used against him.'

I volunteered a bit of his background, how I was sure his mental health had changed due to his time in the army and the unfortunate events life had thrown at him. I told him that the car in question had been given to Paul by his father, so Paul had in fact smashed up his own car. However, I was told that didn't make any difference – he had destroyed something in a rage in a public place, a chargeable offence.

He was instructed to pay his father £5 a week in compensation up to the value of the damage done to the car and, although I believe he paid some of it, it was, to my knowledge, never paid in full. I don't think his father ever complained about not getting all the money. It was left at that but it was clear, as far as both were concerned, the relationship was irredeemably broken and they never made any effort to contact each other again.

After crashing on Steve's sofa overnight, Paul was accompanied by the police back to his father's house the next day so that he could collect some belongings, but it was impossible to take everything. What affected Paul the most was he couldn't find his irreplaceable Red Book from the army, which had always been in the same place but had now disappeared. The book documented all he had achieved with the army, a bit like a CV. He had no time to look for it and with what little he could carry in his rucksack once again, he found himself having to make a quick exit with more or less the clothes he had on his back. All over the price of a drink. He had left what was the only roof over his head; however, he wanted to stay in that area where he knew people.

Paul told me he felt hopeless as he tried to figure out what to do after that unfortunate episode. I can see that many would regard him as a physically healthy young man whose temper hadn't made life easy. Here he was, yet again, making use of his friends' sofas, looking for a low-level job, or trying to claim some form of benefit in a slow and confusing system. In the end, he had enough to rent a room and so he agreed to share a flat with two girls who were friends of friends.

When he called, he told me about his situation, so I suggested I could drive down to visit him in his latest shared accommodation. I didn't know what he owned, so I took a quilt, some towels and, of all things, a wooden ashtray. He was over the moon. His situation prompted me to buy him a few more things, but when I saw his room, he seemed to be coping with what little he had. He also implied he didn't know if he really wanted to stay there. He was quite despondent and said he had nothing much to show for all his time in the army. We touched on him coming to stay with me for a while, but we both knew it wouldn't have worked. I couldn't afford to keep a growing young man for any length of time and he realised that. Also, I had rented out my principal residence when the university offered me a temporary secondment that included basic accommodation in another city. However, I was delighted that Paul was back in Scotland and hoped I would get the chance to support him in finding work and a place to stay. It wasn't difficult to see that he was hankering after Germany again. I had to wait and see where he ended up.

While I was visiting, I took him out for lunch and he started opening up about how things were for him sharing with the girls. He was feeling a bit low, not sleeping and he had a slight medical issue; he thought he had a hernia that he didn't know how to cope with. By the end of the day, I'd taken him to a local doctor for an emergency appointment. He was asked to fill in a form but that seemed to be a huge issue for him. Paul needed help with everyday admin. Many of the questions required answers that he was reluctant to provide. Between us we persevered and got the form filled in, he saw the doctor and he was to be referred to the hospital. He was getting somewhere. Once again I crossed my fingers in the hope that we could beat these physical and mental health concerns.

Over coffee back at the flat, he opened up more and admitted he wasn't all that happy and didn't know how long he'd be able to share accommodation. He said that he was sure the two girls didn't like him. He sat perched on the edge of his single bed with what can only be described as a haunted look, so I prodded more and discovered that a few days before, Paul had commented to the girls about them not cleaning up in the kitchen.

'They leave their dirty plates lying with bits of leftover food all over the worktop. I can't even start to make myself something to eat. They sit and listen to music or go out for hours and I'm fed up having to move stuff,' he complained to me.

'Oh dear,' I whispered. 'Are they home just now?'

'No, this is the day they go home to their family for food and to get their washing done.'

I felt for him. The girls had the benefit of family caring for them; he didn't. I wanted to be more of a mum, his carer, his rock. If he hadn't been sitting in front of me I would have put my head in my hands and wept at his situation. But I couldn't. I couldn't become emotional; we had to find a way forward. A practical approach to getting him back on track.

He interrupted my thoughts by telling me how he had decided to address the kitchen situation a few days beforehand. Regrettably, the girls were dismissive of his complaint and, without wanting to get into an altercation, Paul had eventually gone to his room and fallen asleep. Shortly afterwards, he was awakened by the sound of a vacuum cleaner, which he claimed was right outside his bedroom door, switched on but not moving. He said the girls had deliberately left it running there for hours so that he couldn't sleep. I asked where the girls were while the vacuum cleaner was roaring outside his door, and apparently, they were in the living room, laughing. I wondered how he could hear them if the noise of the machine was so deafening right outside his door. Also, by my calculations, this must have gone on into the small hours of the morning, which didn't make sense.

I questioned him, 'Why didn't you go out and switch it off, or at least ask them what was going on?'

'I tried to, but the door had been wedged shut or locked in some way and I couldn't get out,' he replied. 'I called them but they didn't hear me, or maybe they did but thought it would be funny to leave me stuck in here.'

I made a request. 'Show me how it opens normally.'

Paul easily opened the door. There was no lock and it was difficult to see how he could have been trapped. In my mind, I tried to visualise the situation and wondered what I would have done had it been me locked in. There was a window in the room but, although he was on the ground floor, there was quite a drop to the grass outside. I asked him about getting out that way but he dismissed it, saying he wouldn't have been sure the girls would have let him in if he had knocked on the front door. Then he wouldn't have been able to climb up to get through the window again.

There was something wrong with this story and it pointed to Paul having heard noises that weren't there and somehow mismanaging a door handle or imagining he'd tried to open the door. He said he'd gone back to bed and eventually fallen asleep again. In the morning the door opened without a problem and there was no vacuum cleaner to be seen. Paul and the girls never spoke about it.

He eventually threw into the conversation that he was thinking about going back to Germany. So it looked as though he'd be out of there soon, but I wasn't comfortable with his state of mind. It was hard to tell if he was extremely unsettled because of what had taken place at his father's and maybe a change of scenery would make all the difference to him. Whether or not the girls were concerned about some of his behaviour and wanted him to leave, I never knew. In the end, he left the area but sadly, hadn't stayed there long enough to collect the letter with his much-needed hospital appointment.

Over the next couple of years, he was back and forth between Germany and the UK and I saw and heard from him sporadically. He would take the cheapest form of transport and hitch lifts the rest of the way. Being absent for a while meant that he felt he could arrive as a visitor at someone's door and be pretty sure of a bed for a couple of nights. He did everything on a budget and felt the stress of not knowing where or if he belonged.

It saddened me when he eventually revealed there were times when he wondered if life was worth living. I didn't know then, but in Germany, he spent time with a group of people who had powerful motorbikes. One evening, they were in a large clearing testing out how fast the bikes would go. Paul didn't have a bike but talked someone into lending him one for a test drive. Once he got on the bike and revved it up, he felt some surge of power take over and drove the bike like a maniac without caring what might happen to him or the bike. He never told any of the others, but secretly, he had hoped he would end his life that day.

Between what might have been the near-drowning experience with the army and now this about the motorbike, I was convinced that tempting fate hadn't been a worry to Paul.

Paul had visited us in Scotland at Christmas 1997 and we enjoyed some quality time together. However, I challenged him when I overheard him attempting to make a telephone call to Germany from Cait's flat without asking permission or making any effort to pay. I reminded him who was paying the bill because, being twenty-three, I felt he should have been polite enough to offer. Afterwards, I went into the kitchen, unaware that he and Cait were having a conversation in the bedroom. When she came back through, she told me that Paul had left the flat in a rage with his rucksack; he was gone and wasn't coming back. Cait continued by telling me that he had been furious at me treating him like a child, so much so that he could easily commit suicide. He had hinted at having a gun with him just in case he needed to carry out his threat, a very worrying situation if his story was true. It was gut-wrenching to hear this, as only three months previously a very close family member had taken his own life. We were still reeling from that and it was confusing as to why Paul would allude to such an action knowing the effect it had had on all of us, him included. I didn't think I had the resolve to cope with another tragedy. By then it was about 10 pm and we were worried.

After sitting around for about an hour wondering what to do, we contacted the police who said they'd look out for him at railway and bus stations. We spent a restless night wondering if he was walking the streets, sleeping in a doorway or lying in a ditch.

The police couldn't find him.

The next day, Cait found his friend Steve's number. We thought it highly unlikely that Paul had travelled more than a hundred miles overnight to his friend, but Steve might have been able to give us a clue to his whereabouts. Although I could only hear one side of the conversation, I gathered that not only had he heard from Paul but also he was, at that moment, having a bath in Steve's house.

What I heard next from Cait to Steve chilled me to the bone. She said, 'Can you please pass on a message to Paul? Tell him that we will never be in touch with him again!'

Then she hung up.

She was angry that he had left us worried for hours, but I felt it was a brutal response to finding out he was safe. And her words implied that 'we' included me.

Cait had ended the phone call before any of us could speak to Paul. I missed the opportunity to make amends and clear up the misunderstanding. At least I knew he was safe and that I, for one, would somehow try to get in touch with him again.

He had left without saying goodbye and I guessed he had hitched a lift further south, ending up at one of the few doors he knew would be open to him. I realised Paul was furious with me and I decided not to bug him but to wait until we had both calmed down, hoping that, despite the harsh message from Cait, he would get in touch over the next few days.

The days turned into weeks, then months and, given Paul's tendency to roam, I didn't know where to look for him. I hoped he'd kept my phone number. If Paul didn't want me at this point in his life, I was prepared to accept the situation. I would have felt better if I'd known he was safe and that he had found someone who cared enough to support him and any challenging issues he might be facing. I didn't know how I could find him again, but happily, we were eventually brought together, even if it was under the strangest of circumstances.

BOOK TWO

Chapter 7

News

Unfortunately, the months turned into years and I felt there was something more to Paul's disappearance that I didn't know about. There wasn't any communication between him and Cait, and I carried guilt for not trying to resolve the situation. I often wondered what had happened along the way to make him think I wouldn't want to hear from him again. This was how things were left and four years were to pass before I heard any more about him. It was only when the next part of the story unfolded I realised the incredible dilemma he faced that Christmas in 1997, when he walked out of his sister's flat.

Paul wasn't far from my thoughts over those four years. However, I got through life and found a new job in higher education. After a birthday treat to California to visit a lifelong friend, I threw myself into my lecturing post. I was in the north of Scotland, close to the university, and living on campus which suited me perfectly. I had basic accommodation, but I was in a rewarding job. All that was missing in my life was news of Paul.

When I answered my mobile phone one frosty November day after work, a voice asked if I could identify myself and asked if I was the mother of Paul. I was taken aback. When I told the caller that's exactly who I was, she asked if I was alone. I was and, although she told me she knew she shouldn't deliver certain kinds of news to people who were on their own, she told me she was calling from the Foreign Office in London and that they'd been trying to locate me for a few days. I don't know how they got my mobile phone number, but I guess that's the way things work at higher levels.

She told me that Paul, now twenty-seven, was in Germany. A hospital there had been in touch with them. Apparently, he'd been shot – but was still alive. She could only give me limited information surrounding the incident but, realising I wouldn't be taking everything in, she gave me a number to call first thing the next morning. There are no words for the mix of emotions I felt. My head reeled as I tried to get a picture of Paul; I sat, frozen, letting some of what I'd been told sink in.

Words kept coming and going in my head. *Shot? Why? Still alive? How badly is he hurt?*

Shortly after the call ended, I tidied up and did some ironing, strange behaviour after what I had been told. I think at the back of my mind I knew I'd be going away, possibly for a while, so I wanted to get things in order.

For various reasons, this was a unique time in my life. Practically everyone had been removed from me; the support system that I might otherwise have wished for didn't exist. Perhaps it was destiny that was later to work in my favour. Cait and her partner John, now engaged, were living in another country, my partner had passed away and those who had been soulmates were no longer close. Other family members were either ill or elderly and were dealing with their own circumstances, and Paul's father was completely out of the picture. The situation that was facing me was one I had to deal with on my own.

After the mundane chores had been completed, I called my boss to explain the phone call and to ask for time off. He asked if I'd be OK to come in the next day so that he could help me arrange travel. Early the next morning, I spoke with one of my senior colleagues. As I sat, pale and shaken, she called the Foreign Office on my behalf and, without prompting, asked all the right questions. And so the story unfolded.

It turned out that Paul had been living in a flat alone, had acquired a handgun and had shot himself. He had shot himself upwards through his chin. The bullet was still lodged in his head. I sat at the other side of her desk listening to the conversation as my eyes became wider and my heart beat faster. The shock of it all was incredible, and I was, once again, frozen in time, waiting for the next bit of news. I wanted to get my jacket back on, throw my bag over my shoulder and get to Germany as fast as I could. I had tunnel vision. I guess I might have been feeling similar to Paul when he got the notion to move, and move fast. Thankfully, it was left to my colleague and the Foreign Office to figure out how I could get over to see him.

There were official procedures involved in relaying the message to Paul that I would like to see him. Eventually, I got word that it was all in order. Before I knew it, a plan was forming. My passport was one hundred and fifty miles away in my main residence as I hadn't seen the need to take it to my temporary accommodation at the university. Thankfully, it was transported to me by a good friend. I met her halfway and she took me to Glasgow airport. My work colleague had also told me that Paul's friend Mark, whom I'd never met, would be waiting for me when I landed in Germany and that he'd drive me directly to Göttingen University Hospital. Throwing a few things in a bag and grabbing some currency, I was ready for my journey.

Apart from the few people who had stepped in at the last minute, I never told another living soul what had happened or where I was going. I needed to know more before I could finally let the family know what had happened and I was to rely on Mark for at least part of the background to this event.

I felt the aeroplane wasn't going quick enough; my thoughts were racing faster than the flight. After three hours, questions were still churning in my head, but by then we had finally landed at the airport in Germany. I had no option but to follow my fellow passengers to the exit. I didn't know the language, and I didn't even know who I was looking for. I felt lost as I scanned the few people waiting for passengers to emerge at arrivals, but soon I saw a tall, fair-haired young man standing as close as he could to the barrier. I hadn't even thought about Paul's surname being on a placard, but Mark had had the foresight to do that. As we introduced ourselves, I realised I wasn't the only one nervous and lost for words.

Walking to his car, I could only keep thanking Mark for meeting me – this was a luxury I very seldom had at airports. He knew where we were going so I could, to a certain extent, sit back. It was a delight to have someone to take the weight of further travel off my shoulders. We drove for over an hour towards Göttingen but I was only half-heartedly taking in the surroundings: everything was written in German, of course, but I must admit to being drawn to the normality of life outside. Feeling completely out of my depth, I had to find out what Paul had been doing for the last four years and how things had come to this. Although Mark was also in shock, I could tell he needed someone to take over the responsibility for Paul. I was tired from travelling but I had a few inquisitive questions; all I asked of Mark was that he told me the truth. I was ready to respect his replies even if he said he'd rather not answer me. I didn't want coverups or lies. He promised he'd tell me everything he knew and began by explaining how he had met Paul.

Mark was one of a small group of five friends that had included Paul. All were about the same age; they had bonded many years ago in Germany. The others were, or had been, soldiers, but not Mark. Nevertheless, he was one of the boys. When they discovered that they were all from broken homes, having experienced turbulent childhoods, they truly united. In the early days of being in the army, Paul had brought some of these friends over to visit Scotland, where they were quick to seek out the nearest nightclub and impress the girls, but Mark hadn't been one of them; they'd met later.

As happens, life had taken them all in different directions as they grew older. Some had steady girlfriends, but they were still a united force, looking out for one another. Paul had returned to Germany after the Christmas he had left us under a cloud, and, once reunited with his group of friends, they had many a good time. However, Paul had barely been back a few months when he told them that he wanted to return to the UK to see his family; whether he intended his visit to be short-term or for good, none of them knew. Mark had been surprised because it seemed as if Paul had only just arrived and now wanted to trail off again. As it was, that was one of many visits he was to make to Scotland over a few years, but Paul always ran short of money after a matter of months and was forced back to Germany. Sadly, he never made any contact with our family in Scotland. Through time, the friends had become concerned about his conduct and appearance.

Paul felt he hadn't been dealt a good hand with jobs and apartments in Germany. There came points where he had exhausted all avenues and that's why he had kept returning to the UK. He was like a train going in and out of tunnels, not knowing what would be at the end of each one. In Germany, he had learned to communicate verbally in the language. Communicating by letter or completing an application form proved to be massive obstacles for him. Even though he would find out about and maybe even secure jobs through friends of friends, he was continually chasing his tail financially. Also, without transport, it was practically impossible to accept work unless it was on his doorstep. Despite not having a regular income, banks and loan companies were enticing him to borrow, which he did. Although there had been some very kind people who took him under their wing and gave him food, a bed and a few coins now and again; these arrangements were unsustainable.

The friends realised Paul was in pretty dire straits financially when he started turning down chances to go out with the group. His appearance was shoddy and he was becoming withdrawn. He had travelled back and forth to the UK hitching lifts. The last time he travelled back to Germany, things had been different according to Mark. Paul was as dishevelled, disorientated and as nervous as when he'd left. He told me Paul had hitched lifts throughout

England but didn't quite make it to Scotland and, within days, had returned to Germany.

As the journey to the hospital continued, Mark also told me that, a few months previously, he was confused by Paul's attitude and it seemed as if he was losing control of his thoughts as well as his finances. Paul had approached Mark to ask for money, not only money to survive for a day or two, but also money to buy a motorbike. No amount was mentioned, only that he wanted enough to buy a motor bike. Taken aback, Mark questioned Paul about this strong notion. He explained that he would be able to take a job further away if he had his own transport. Although that was a logical argument, what wasn't so logical was that Paul didn't have an interview, never mind a job, nor did he have a motorbike licence, and he certainly didn't have the money to tax, insure or fill a bike with fuel. Mark had to refuse him, as nicely as he could, pointing out that he didn't have enough money to give to Paul anyway. He was surprised at Paul's angry reaction at him not supporting the idea. I asked if, hypothetically, he had been able to help Paul, would he have done so?

Mark replied, 'To be honest, I don't think I would have. When he was talking about it he seemed to have a strange, dark and distant look in his eyes. He seemed far away and was quite forceful in his manner.'

He remarked that he had never seen Paul like that before and when Mark had asked him if he knew how much he was asking for, Paul had turned on his heel and left. Mark had been concerned that the incident might have spoiled their friendship; however, the bike was never mentioned again and Paul was his old self the next time they met.

Nevertheless, Mark kept that unusual incident in mind as other things began to develop.

It all went from bad to worse financially for Paul and, eventually, he had no choice but to live in a friend's garden shed for a short while, being given food by the generous family until eventually, it all became too much and he was asked to leave. Somehow, he managed to secure a small apartment but by then he had practically stopped seeing his friends altogether.

About a week before my arrival in Germany, Paul had made a late-night phone call to Mark, mumbling and stumbling over his words. Mark asked him a few times what he was trying to say but eventually put it down to Paul having had a few too many, which in itself surprised him because he knew Paul didn't have any money to buy beer. They hung up eventually. Living a distance away, Mark couldn't easily get to Paul's flat; however, he was haunted through the night by the phone call and first thing next morning he called another friend, Grant, who lived nearer Paul, asking him to pop round and see what was going on. Grant was working that day but promised he would swing by in a day or two.

It was the following day before Grant and his girlfriend eventually knocked on Paul's door. Paul spoke through the closed door and asked Grant if he was alone. When he said he wasn't, Paul said he would let him in but not his girlfriend. Finally, the door opened a fraction and Grant was able to squeeze through. What he saw will probably stay with him forever. He walked into something out of a horror movie. The flat was completely covered in blood: mirrors, carpets and sofa, with the addition of blood-soaked towels strewn around the floors. Paul could hardly stand; he fell back on the sofa and appeared to black out. He had managed to tell Grant that he'd shot himself and that the gun was lying on the table. Grant immediately called the emergency services.

When help first arrived, Paul was lying unconscious. He came round to see the barrels of three police guns trained on him while medics stood by. As some of them searched the flat, the others made frantic calls and prepared him for hospital while trying to keep him conscious. He was strapped onto a gurney and wheeled out to an ambulance which took him to a waiting emergency helicopter. Later I was to learn that he had been desperate for the toilet but couldn't do anything other than keep it in on a helicopter journey that seemed to take forever. He was sure his bladder was about to burst. I thought that should have been the least of his worries.

I asked Mark if Paul had been taking drugs of any kind. He assured me Paul wasn't, that was all history for the young men. He admitted that in the past they'd taken some mood enhancers when they were going out to raves or the Love Parade, a huge event in Germany, but that had long since stopped because both Mark and Grant now had girlfriends and had left their wildest days behind them. He assured me Paul wouldn't have been able to afford drugs anyway. I asked about any romantic relationships but it seemed there had only ever been fleeting encounters; after Dee had broken up with him he'd never really got over her. I appreciated Mark's honesty, but further questions would have to wait as we finally arrived in Göttingen.

Chapter 8

German Hospitality

As Mark had already visited Paul, he knew where to go. We parked up and, as we walked towards the main hospital entrance, I suddenly became overwhelmed and froze on the spot. I asked him if he thought this visit would be OK and if Paul really wanted to see me after all these years.

He looked at me with a smile on his face and said, 'You're his mum. Of course he wants to see you!'

His reassuring words gave me the courage to take the next few steps forward, and the automatic glass doors glided open. Inside the hospital, everything was obviously in German. People milled around, various reception areas were buzzing with people and there was an atmosphere of urgency about the whole place. Patients were being pushed into lifts in wheelchairs and families were sitting in waiting areas. We made our way downstairs. In the basement area, the atmosphere changed as if we had descended into the bowels of the earth; this was where Paul was.

No one was around. Everything was silent, and the door at the bottom of the stairs was locked. Mark pressed a large silver button on the intercom system, but we heard nothing. With no chairs or tables placed at the downstairs entrance to welcome visitors, I would have been forgiven for thinking I was in a factory, but the sterile hospital smell brought me back to reality. We waited like disobedient children until a few minutes later, a man dressed in a pale blue uniform emerged through the locked door. Mark explained, in German, who we were. Satisfied, he led us through yet another set of doors that revealed a long corridor. The pale blue walls seemed to go on forever, as did the dark blue markings on the floor. Off to each side of the prison-like corridor was a series of numbered double doors, which didn't even have the usual small windows partway up. Mark explained that these weren't regular wards – the authorities designed them especially for those who needed security because they could be a danger to themselves or others. The man in pale blue showed us to the correct door and, once through, we found ourselves in a small entrance. I followed Mark's lead. We had to wash our hands with sanitiser and put on shoe covers, as well as blue gowns, before we could enter. Everything was well organised.

The next thing I knew, I was being directed into a single room where I could see someone lying on a bed with their back to me. There were tubes, lines, drips and monitors everywhere. The outline of the pink striped bedcovers showed the form of a body with a mop of unruly hair sprawled out onto a pink striped pillowcase. Despite being in the basement, the room was light. Without curtains or blinds on the windows, the afternoon sun hit the metallic stands that held the bags of liquid medication; the unexpected brightness immediately lifted my spirits.

A movement from the bed revealed a pale-faced Paul who had turned his head around.

'I've been waiting for days for you to come,' he said weakly.

I could only smile at him. 'I'm here now!'

I swear I could feel the inside of my body shaking. I felt dwarfed by the machinery and even somewhat intimidated by the staff who were in and out, checking and replacing, reading charts and writing notes. I had to pull myself together and pray that my trembling wasn't evident. Although full of tension and anxiety, strangely enough, there was an inner peace that I was once again doing my job as a mother, ready to comfort her broken son. I leaned over through all the paraphernalia and kissed Paul's cheek and, as he turned towards me again, I stroked his arm. Mark stayed a short while then left us together. He headed home with the suggestion that we meet again before I left Germany, which was fine by me. After four years I was finally looking at my boy again, and although I had more questions to ask, these could wait.

We passed a few comments but, initially, it was hard to know what to say. An English-speaking doctor joined us and gave me a quick résumé on Paul's condition. Also, he wanted to know how long I'd be staying. Paul was quiet during our chat, never saying a word as the doctor explained the damage caused by the bullet. As I hadn't arranged a place to stay, the doctor told me of a nearby hotel where families of patients usually stayed. That was perfect, as far as I was concerned.

I hadn't been with Paul for more than a quarter of an hour when a smartly dressed deputation of two men and a woman arrived at the bottom of his bed. They spoke in German to both Paul and me, but I didn't understand a word.

Paul uttered a few words to them, then turned to me and, almost under his breath, muttered, 'Don't speak to them, Mum. This is about who pays for me being in here.'

I thought, *He's pretty switched on for someone who's lying with a bullet in his head!*

I turned to the English-speaking doctor. 'Please, could you ask them to give me some time alone with my son? I've just arrived from Scotland and I've got all I can deal with at the moment.'

He translated and the little group nodded and moved away. To clear things up, Paul told me he had the official documentation that allowed him medical cover in Germany. The doctor explained that, as Paul hadn't been in a fit state to produce any paperwork, the authorities thought he was a holidaymaker or someone who had recently arrived in the country. If that had been the case, unlike in the UK with the NHS available to all, they would have expected him to have private medical insurance or that some family member would foot the bill. As it was, Paul had already registered with the German healthcare system so, when I was armed with his ID number, I could sort this out for him. I was relieved, as the extra cost of paying for a helicopter would certainly have stretched my budget.

Paul, however, was not as alert as I'd initially thought. He was dazed, although now and again he was speaking sense. Even as I sat at his bedside, he would close his eyes, probably not sleeping soundly but maybe in a dreamlike state, relieved and relaxed that someone was there with him. When his eyes were closed, I looked closer at my surroundings. My breathing almost stopped as I tried to take in all that was in the room: oversized screens and large computer towers, smaller pieces of medical monitoring equipment and lots of beeping noises. One screen displayed three columns, which were highlighted in red, blue or yellow. I wouldn't have understood what it all meant even if the words had been in English – it looked very technical and overwhelming.

After a quick survey of the room, I looked again at the bed where Paul lay. I looked closer at the tubes and the different coloured connections that came from beneath the covers and led to somewhere under the bed. He was calm but I noticed the pillow was starting to work its way out of the pink striped pillowcase, which was an indication to me that he must have had a restless period. One pillow was massive, more akin to a floor cushion. I wondered if this was standard in German hospitals or if there was a reason – maybe he needed to be propped up. Insignificant thoughts like this popped up as I tried to internalise my surroundings. When he opened his eyes, the usual questions surfaced but were kept firmly in my head. I wanted to ask, *What have you done to yourself? What were you thinking?*

I knew what he'd done, I didn't need to ask. And asking what he had been thinking would have sounded like a scolding.

I suppose my most pertinent silent thought was, *There's a bullet inside this head that I'm looking at.*

It seemed bizarre, but I noticed an insignificant detail on the duvet cover – Göttingen 1995 was interwoven into the pattern. That was the year when Paul had decided he'd had enough of army life and told them he was leaving. When the cover was being manufactured, he was surely hoping for a life that certainly wouldn't involve lying under that very piece of linen.

After an hour, I had to leave to check into the hotel but promised Paul I'd be back very soon. I asked what the plastic bag was beside his bed and he told me it contained the clothes he had been wearing when he had been brought in. I suggested I take them and wash them; I think he would have agreed to anything at that moment. I had been told the wounds to his mouth and throat meant he wouldn't be able to eat or have regular mealtimes; he was being drip-fed so I was free to visit anytime.

The hotel room was on the second floor, a typical basic room, clean and tidy with a spacious bathroom and a neat pile of towels. I wasn't intending to spend much time there so I unpacked the few items I'd brought from Scotland then looked at the bag I'd brought from the hospital. I didn't know exactly what was inside; I felt as though I was sneaking a look at someone else's property. I tentatively emptied everything into the bathroom sink. Paul's clothes fell out: a pair of jeans, some underwear and a casual shirt. No jumper, no jacket, no personal belongings. Everything was covered in blood, the jeans and the shirt more so than the rest. I filled the bath and made lather out of some shampoo. Then I washed the least affected items first before hanging them over the bath taps. Next, I tackled the jeans.

Within seconds of being submerged in fresh water and suds, blood started to seep out. My son's blood, lots of blood from the body I had given life to; not like blood from a scraped knee or split lip. The white foam drank in the red and the water turned pink. I shook my head as I thought about what must have been in Paul's mind, and the poor mothers whose children don't survive such trauma. I had no option but to continue filling and emptying the water again and again until it ran clear. With nowhere to wring or dry the jeans, I had to hang them over the shower head; their presence and the monotonous drip a continual reminder of what had happened.

Over the next week, I got things in order. As long as I could rest at night, I was able to spend my time at the hospital. For the first couple of days, Paul kept falling asleep and could neither sit up nor focus to read for any length of time. I couldn't buy him food or drink; I couldn't give him anything but my presence. He was extremely paranoid during that time, watching everyone who passed by with suspicion and convincing himself he was being fed antifreeze. He whispered that he could see a blue liquid inside one of the bags attached to a tube. When the nurse came in, I asked what was in the bags and she explained that, because Paul couldn't have anything by mouth, he was being tube-fed nutrition; other bags were for medication and to hydrate him. To try and convince Paul he was not being given antifreeze, I asked her about the colour and told her we thought one was blue. She looked at it from different angles but didn't see what he saw; she suggested it might be a strange reflection from the sun coming through the window. This didn't appease Paul, he was still doubtful and shook his head slightly to indicate that I shouldn't believe her.

My days were spent either sitting by his bedside or grabbing a snack in the hospital canteen. Even though he would drift in and out of sleep, I wanted to stay by his side – to show him his life mattered. Bit by bit, I began to piece together what had happened. The bullet had gone up through his chin and damaged the roof of his mouth and part of his throat. It had then travelled up behind his nose and his eyes but there was no exit wound. It was lodged in one side of his head and he needed an operation to remove it. The medical staff also realised that he was in grave need of counselling and they were trying to figure out which of Paul's needs was the most urgent.

Initially, the staff told me they would give Paul some psychiatric help, after which they would remove the bullet. The reason for his mental issues being addressed first was because the operation would be a tricky procedure, and they were struggling to find a surgeon who was willing to perform it. Into the bargain, after a couple of days of ongoing tests, we got the disturbing news that Paul had contracted bacterial meningitis that, if not treated, could be deadly. Two things contributed to this: first that he had made the bullet from bits of metal that were lying around and probably dirty, and second that it had travelled up the back of his throat, carrying bacteria with it. Although the bullet had to be taken out, he couldn't have an operation until the infection was treated and settled. With these obstacles preventing surgery, it made sense that the psychiatric appointment would take priority once Paul felt up to it.

Lying in bed he seemed physically OK but, one day before I visited, he had asked if he could get up to have a shower. After being helped to the shower area, he was insistent that he would manage the rest himself. He had turned on the tap when he felt his legs give way. He hadn't even hit the ground before the shower door was flung open and two members of staff were there to help him back to bed. Much weaker than he thought, he duly followed orders and stayed put until the next day.

From his hospital bed, he began telling me he'd made both the gun and the bullet himself from bits and pieces he had acquired. Although he freely spoke about what had happened, I convinced him we could speak about the finer details at a later date. He had to pull through this first. Eventually, I was allowed to take him out of his room in a wheelchair, but only within the confines of the locked ground floor. That meant pushing him up and down the corridor, where he could get his bearings and see what was going on in the rooms nearby.

Above his bed was a sign in German, translated it read, 'Nil by Mouth'. Other patients could eat, and the smell of cooked food was frustrating Paul. Outside the rooms, trolleys with leftover bits of breakfast, lunch or dinner waited to be removed. He mentioned he would gladly devour anything that was there. We joked about it and, as I pushed the wheelchair past a waiting trolley, he stretched an arm out, pretending to take an unopened tub of yoghurt. My heart flipped, and I nearly crashed the wheelchair into the wall, trying to divert it away from the leftover food. He might have died if he'd tried to swallow anything.

He turned his head around as far as he could to see my face and joked, 'Got you there, eh?'

His room was bare, with no cards, no water or fruit. The usual bits and pieces that often litter a patient's bedside cabinet were missing. Within the main hospital, there were a few small shops and I spotted one that sold magazines and postcards. Everything was in German. I found a postcard of a doctor's consulting room where an extremely short-sighted doctor with overly thick glasses was sitting behind his desk. A patient was on the other side of the desk, holding his decapitated head under his arm. I had to ask the shop assistant to translate what the doctor on the postcard was saying. It read, 'And so my friend, what seems to be the problem?' I knew that was the card for Paul. The irony of no one being able to see what was going on in his life and him trying to shoot his head off would not have been lost on him. I wrote a message on the postcard but, before I handed it over, I spoke with the member of staff in charge to ask if I was taking it a step too far with this kind of humour.

He laughed as he announced, 'Absolutely not. Paul will love that!'

I believed that this particular man had somehow seen through Paul's attempt to take his own life and had recognised that underneath there was a young man who had another side to him.

In time, Paul spoke about the night he had caused himself this near-fatal injury. He thought that one way to solve his problems was with a gun.

Chapter 9

No Way Out

It was clear that a pattern had emerged where, if Paul felt backed into a corner, he would run, disappear, making sure he was difficult to find. He told me he was sure he had burned his bridges in Scotland and had all but exhausted the generosity of friends in Germany. The time had come when he had nowhere to run, nowhere to hide and no one to turn to. He had no money, he was hungry and he was out of options.

As we sat opposite each other in the small hospital room, he was able to raise a wry smile as he recounted, 'It was all because of pasta.'

I screwed my eyes up, thinking he'd been served pasta somewhere and it had given him a bad stomach. 'Eh? What about pasta?'

'One day last week, I began to get hungry around one o'clock. I knew there wasn't much in the cupboard but when I looked in I saw a jar of pickles and some sugar. The only thing to eat, the only thing to make a meal with, was pasta, and I didn't feel like pasta. It had been there for ages and I didn't have any sauce anyway. I'd finished everything else so I closed the cupboard door.'

I teased, 'Hoping for a miracle that it might multiply like the loaves and the fishes?'

Quick as a flash he came back with, 'No, that would only have meant more pasta! Didn't want that!' He continued, 'It was that thick tube kind of pasta. Nobody can eat that without sauce. But the strange thing was, I kept going back to open the cupboard door.' He made fun of the fact that he would open the door and peer round to see if it was still there, tormenting him.

But there was a serious side to this – he realised all this had to end. Something had snapped. I had to surmise that this wasn't all to do with a packet of pasta. It was about losing everything and everyone; it was about feeling helpless with nowhere to turn.

He told the story as if it had happened to someone else, someone in a very different frame of mind. That day, with nothing much left in his life, he focused on what he felt he was good at; assembling bits and pieces as he had done as a boy, but this time he was making a gun and some bullets. It took him hours and, when he was finished, he sat down to admire his handiwork. Then, with the gun in his hand, he got up, stood in front of his mirror, put the barrel under his chin and pulled the trigger. Nothing happened. He adjusted it and tried again. Nothing. He made yet another adjustment and tried again. It worked.

He remembered that the bang was deafening. All he could hear was buzzing in his ears as he stood for a few seconds looking into the mirror before involuntarily falling back onto the sofa. He told me things appeared to happen in slow motion. The gun fell to the floor, although he couldn't hear it drop because of the buzzing sound. Something wet dripped onto his arm. He looked; it was red, it was blood.

More blood started pouring out from his chin. His first thought was to get to the bathroom for a towel or something. He initially tried to stand up, but his head was reeling and he couldn't get his legs to take his weight. After what seemed like an eternity, he started to crawl, making a blood trail similar to that of a wounded animal trying to escape from a predator. Partway there, he eased himself up by holding onto an armchair, then stumbled to the bathroom. He got a towel and managed to get back to the sofa but blacked out again. When he came round, the buzzing had stopped and there was much more blood on the floor. He carefully bent over, lifted the gun and placed it on the coffee table.

He had said to himself, *Well, at least that worked!*

Trying to steady himself again, he made his way to collect more towels, sheets… anything to stem the flow of blood.

He was in and out of consciousness for hours and then days, never knowing night from day, only that somehow it became easier to move around. He even had a shower. His mouth and throat were on fire and all he could think about as he lay down was how he would love the coolness of an ice lolly to chill his burning throat and quench his maddening thirst. He didn't know it then but, luckily, he hadn't damaged his tongue, which must have rolled back in his mouth when the gun finally fired.

The normal fight, flight and freeze responses were coming and going for me. To some extent, I wanted to fight the gun away from him, but it was too late for that. I wanted to grab him, get him out of the situation as he lay wounded, but that moment had passed. I was helpless because the deed was done. I could only sit, rooted to the spot and listen as though I were in a cinema where a riveting film was capturing my every sense. Wild horses could not have dragged me from my physical or mental state. The moment where shock meets disbelief created a blind spot and, rather than Paul's words filtering in at a manageable pace, my brain switched between slow motion and fast forward. I knew I might have to ask him to repeat what he had just told me so that I could process it logically.

While this incredible story was unfolding from his hospital bed, I could see Paul's sense of humour had remained; I asked him what he did to get some relief from the burning in his mouth.

He joked, 'Well, I tried to have a drink of water, but it ran out of the hole in my chin!'

Humour aside, this was a great deal to take in. So much had happened in such a brief space of time with such disastrous results that often the chronological order of events didn't register with me immediately. It was clear, though, that this was the same as the other times he had wanted to get away and leave everything, only this time he was prepared to leave life itself behind.

I needed to go back home to sort some things out and, given the delay with the operation, I decided after a week to go and set a few wheels in motion with doctors, social services and such like in Scotland. I was intending to come back to Germany to be with Paul until all the treatments were over and he had the all-clear. Then he would come home with me.

I said goodbye to Paul and made the surreal trip back home. When I woke up in my bed the next morning I had to pinch myself – I couldn't believe what the previous week had uncovered. Only seven days before I had wakened in the same bed never realising what lay behind the call from the Foreign Office. Now I wanted to pave the way for Paul's return while trying to keep some normality in my daily work life.

Once I had caught up on sleep, I got in touch with some family and friends to tell them what had happened. I made visits as quickly as I could and tried to break the news without putting the fear of death into them while gauging their reactions face to face. It wasn't a problem to tell them I had found out Paul was in hospital in Germany recovering from a gunshot wound; the conversation stopper was when I explained that he had shot himself. I felt that was enough and the details behind how he made the gun and the four days he lay bleeding could wait. I decided I would avoid burdening folk with updates if that wasn't what they wanted and, once he was back, I could dissuade contact between Paul and anyone I detected would feel uncomfortable with him.

It was only when I saw reactions first-hand that I realised the battle we might face. I cried many a night as I remembered some of the conversations. I was told to leave him in Germany where he was, that he would use up all my time, energy and money, forever. Some folk were afraid and worried about what they should do if he turned up at their door, and more or less told me to keep him away. Others thought he should be locked up because he would never fully be a part of our family again and wouldn't be invited to be part of whatever we were doing.

Sadly, I couldn't tell Paul that everyone was waiting to welcome him but that didn't mean *I* had to disconnect from him. He was still my son and the last thing I wanted was to see him backed into a corner again and made to feel like an outcast. I felt he was worth saving. As I saw it, he was a tortured soul trying to deal with a difficult life. With few people behind me, I was more or less on my own, but not for long. Paul was coming back and hopefully soon.

Every evening, I was able to call Paul at the hospital and get an update. We chatted for about half an hour each time and I told him how I was progressing with, for example, social services. Then, on day three, he said he had some news. The meningitis had cleared and they had found a female surgeon who was willing to operate and remove the bullet. The plan was to take some skin from the top of his leg to repair the inside of his throat, chin and mouth, then, possibly two or three days later, to carry out the more intricate operation to extract the bullet. These procedures were to start immediately, the next day in fact, and so the appointment with the psychiatrist was put on hold.

I could have dropped everything there and then and gone back over to Germany but he talked me out of it, saying that there was no point because he'd likely be sleeping for days after the operation. I called the ward the next afternoon but could only speak to the staff, who assured me the skin grafts had gone according to plan and that Paul was resting. We spoke the following day and he was upbeat until he told me that if anything went wrong the next day while they were trying to remove the bullet, he didn't want to be kept alive on a machine.

I started to ask him, 'What do you expect me to —?'

'Switch it off,' he interrupted.

That was a long, worrying day for me and no doubt a testing time for Paul. We were in different countries doing very different things. I looked at the clock on my office wall – it was 9 am on the dot, 10 am in Germany, and the time of reckoning. I imagined him being prepped for the operation; hair shaved and a sterile gown. He hadn't sounded unduly worried the day before but, with a serious operation only minutes away, he must have wondered if he would see the light of day again. I couldn't help thinking that death was what he had wanted only days before and prayed that he now was ready to grasp life again. I watched the minutes tick by and closed my eyes now and again to focus on sending positive vibes.

I never asked how long the operation had taken when I called the ward later in the day; it was enough to know the decision about switching off a lifesaving machine was one I didn't have to make – the bullet had been successfully removed. Paul was out of theatre, now awake but resting. I was assured I could speak to him later.

Paul had been moved from the secure ward post-op and was sharing a room with another patient. When I called the first couple of times, it was difficult for him to hear me because he had what he called a cage around his head to protect his wound. He couldn't put the phone close to his ear. I was encouraged when, despite his physical injuries and mental condition, he was concerned about the welfare of his roommate. His companion, a young man, had a tumour on his brain and wasn't sure if the operation he had undergone had been successful. They were both patients with different perspectives on life and yet had been brought together under such tragic circumstances. Paul was discharged before he found out whether or not his companion survived.

I learned that, on leaving the hospital, he asked the doctor if he could please have the bullet back. He was given a resounding, 'No!'

However, they gave him two photographs of the bullet next to a ruler, which showed its size, around 2cm long.

They decided not to give Paul any psychiatric help but to discharge him and let him go back to his own country as soon as possible. The wheels were now turning in our favour; he could come back and build a life in Scotland. However, as is always the way in life, there were a few obstacles to overcome first.

The last time I had seen him in Scotland was when he had left us wondering where he had disappeared to so late at night. Eventually, he filled the gaps about that fateful December.

Chapter 10

Lost Years

When he left at Christmas time four years previously, there were few possibilities open to Paul. Eventually, he gave me an account of the direction his life had taken. He was sure his sister and I didn't want to be in touch with him again – after all, and whether it was true, that Christmas evening he'd told Cait he had a gun with him and complained he was being treated like a child. They spoke some harsh words in anger between them, but I didn't hear nor appreciate the seriousness of the situation. All I had cared about was Paul's happiness and, if that meant him leaving and staying away from us, then that was how it would need to be. With his father no longer in the picture, he felt it was impossible to go anywhere near family. I discovered he had hitched different lifts until he arrived at Steve's house. Crashing on a sofa was something he could do with friends for a few nights.

After reflecting on his situation, he left Scotland and, with very little money, hitchhiked again but this time he managed to find a way to cross the Channel. From the ferry windows he watched and said goodbye to the UK, then soon felt relief at seeing the familiar sights of the countryside and towns on the other side. He got through Europe and felt he was reaching his goal, especially when the road signs and shop fronts indicated he was on German soil. Naturally, old friends welcomed him with open arms and rallied round as best they could to help him slip back into the simple lifestyle that he was accustomed to. In time, he secured a couple of part-time jobs, which gave him a bit of money. However, with no permanent or consistent employment, there was no security; very quickly he was back to square one.

Paul had always been particular about his appearance, especially his hair, preferring to be clean and smart rather than looking like something the cat had dragged in. To continue to be presentable under such conditions was difficult. Living from hand to mouth with very few clothes or extra money even to spend on a haircut, he became despondent. Drifting between low-end jobs, he found himself again in an environment where he could be duped by unscrupulous employers but without recourse to complain. Waiting for payments that never appeared or working extra hours without being paid an overtime rate, made him feel angry and powerless. To me, it was clear that his mental health must have continued to suffer under these conditions. Some people thrive by being spontaneous and taking opportunities, others sink because they move on impulse. In my opinion, Paul was impulsive. He would jump into a situation without thinking through the consequences. I didn't understand mental health issues but I could see that life was all a bit of a gamble for him, in which there were winners and losers. If he won, like everyone else he was on top of the world, but if he lost or things didn't work out, he didn't have coping strategies. The downward spiral of his mental state would begin manifesting in irrational thinking, apportioning blame and turning away from others. These were traits that, thinking back, mirrored some of his childhood experiences.

Mark had already told me the last journey Paul had made between Germany and the UK was one that had left his friends worried. Now Paul could shed some light on his demeanour at that time. One morning, he was ironing a pair of jeans, wondering what to make of his life. He stopped what he was doing to listen to the British Prime Minister, Tony Blair, who was delivering a speech on German TV. Partway through, he heard Blair speaking directly to him. The PM announced that people were out to get Paul; they knew he was in Germany and he needed to make his way back to the UK if he wanted to stay safe. Bizarrely, he decided to follow these instructions; he thought maybe this was a sign that he should try to contact his family in the UK, that the time had come to build bridges. Paul said goodbye to the kind people in Germany who had, yet again, given him the necessities of life when he most needed them. When his friends commented on how shabby he was becoming, he joked with them that he was trying to look more like a hippy-type traveller.

With nothing much on his person, he got through France between buses and hitchhiking and over to a port in the south of England. He wanted to get straight to London, where he could rest and make plans for the next leg of his journey up to Scotland. He was dishevelled. His hair was long, greasy and unkempt, his body was filthy and his clothes and shoes were shabby. He had nothing but a few belongings that he carried in a plastic bag; he had nowhere to go in London. He was embarrassed to say that he started begging for a little money as soon as he arrived.

With downcast eyes, he admitted, 'I asked a few guys at the port if they could spare some coins. A couple of them did and I bought a cup of tea and a plate of chips. I learned to ask folk who were on their own.'

I mentioned that I didn't know what I'd do if someone asked me for money. I knew I would be afraid to bring out my purse in case it was snatched.

'Ah well, you learn who to ask, and beggars don't usually ask women for money.' He never gave me a reason but his explanation clarified why I'd never been asked for money by anyone in the street. I can only imagine the number of people who would have swerved away from him as he approached them. However, he had finally made it to the PM's territory.

That first night in London, Paul was tired but couldn't find anywhere for him and his plastic bag to go. He walked around well into the small hours of the morning. With no particular place in mind, he caught a few hours' sleep on a park bench until he heard unfamiliar accents speaking. It took him a minute or two to come round, only to discover two English policemen towering over him.

'Wake up. You can't sleep here, it's not allowed. Where are you from?'

Paul didn't want to divulge anything; he was steeped in the pattern of thinking that everyone was out to get him, so he mumbled something between German and English before saying he was just about to move on anyway.

They told him that he'd be arrested if he lay there and waited until he walked away. He walked for miles, stopping now and again if he got the chance to rest on some steps. Finally, he found another bench where he could sit for a while.

His face strained as he continued, 'By this time, my feet were really sore. I had to take my shoes and socks off to look. Both feet were swollen and covered in blisters and, into the bargain, I could only hobble as the sole of one trainer was parting company with the rest.'

As if things weren't bad enough.

Throughout the day, he tried to get his bearings as he wandered around asking for some coins and grabbing a cup of tea when he could. On the second night, he was not happy about sleeping in a doorway or under a bridge, and he didn't want to risk a park bench again. When he came across a quiet, tree-lined street where one tree had thick branches, he reckoned he had found the perfect place to hide where perhaps he could shut his eyes for a few hours.

After surveying the area and assuring himself that no one could see him clearly through the dusk of the evening, he climbed the tree to the widest branch and carefully balanced himself, holding on with one hand to see if he could reach higher with his other. He reached up and carefully hid the plastic bag on the branch above, where it couldn't be seen from the ground. Uncomfortable as he was, he managed to get some sleep and in the early hours, he wakened to the sound of birds chirping, demonstrably annoyed at their unwelcome visitor. Paul jumped down.

Not knowing the area, he kept walking along the unfamiliar streets until he came across someone or something. Suddenly, he realised he'd left his plastic bag up the tree. He turned to look at where he'd been and quickly made it back to the first corner, but he'd no idea which direction he'd come from. He glanced down a few quiet side streets, but they all looked alike. He looked up at the trees but, in the cold light of day, these all looked the same too.

He knew he had hidden the bag so well that even if he were standing right under the actual tree, he wouldn't be able to see it. He had to abandon his search and leave the plastic bag behind.

With nowhere to go, he told himself this was all the fault of the PM, who had suggested he come back to the UK for safety. He firmly believed that his dilemma had been created yet again because of the *system* and the way governments ran their countries.

Now that he had lost his belongings, all he had was an old watch on his wrist and a worn, practically empty wallet in his pocket. The wallet was sacred because it shielded a few of his German friends' phone numbers and his passport. Armed with his remaining possessions, he made his way to 10 Downing Street and asked the policeman on the gate if he could speak to Tony Blair. Of course, his request was refused and so after taking his watch off, he asked if it could be passed on to the PM.

The policeman responded, 'There is no facility for that type of thing to happen.'

So Paul placed the watch on the ground in front of the police officer and announced, 'He's taken everything else of mine, so he might as well have this.'

As he walked away, he realised the excruciating pain from the blisters on his feet meant he couldn't carry on much further. When he passed a sign that read, *Doctor*, Paul went in. He didn't care what kind of doctor he would find inside; he only wanted to ask someone to tend to his feet. He must have looked a fright because he told me that a few waiting people looked at him wide-eyed as he demanded to see someone immediately. A doctor appeared and took him into the surgery then asked him a few questions. He washed

Paul's feet, creamed and bandaged them. While he was attending to Paul, the doctor gave him some advice about where he might go for some support. Not thinking logically and already distressed, the doctor's suggestions were too much for Paul to cope with, but at least he walked out in a better condition than he went in.

He had the idea of heading to a transport café to hitch a lift to Scotland and walked along to a service station with trucks lined up outside. That convinced him his luck was in as he thought, *Surely one driver will help me?*

One area of the café seemed to be designated for the drivers so he spoke with a group sitting around a couple of tables. Unfortunately, none of the men were driving to Scotland. Paul told them his story of coming from Germany and needing to get in touch with his family, so one driver agreed to take him partway. The driver was heading home to the Newcastle area, just short of Scotland, after his last delivery. As a delighted Paul jumped into the cab, they set off on their five-hour journey. Stopping off halfway at yet another transport café, the kind driver bought Paul a snack and a cup of tea before they carried on. Although they made small talk during their time together, Paul was reluctant to trust the man with too much detailed information. The driver said he would only spend one night at home with his wife before he had to retrace his steps and head back down south again. He offered to arrange an onward lift for Paul, but that wouldn't happen until the following day. After his delivery, he kindly suggested that Paul stay with him and his wife that night. He told Paul he would get something to eat; he could also have a bath and a good night's sleep. Despite sounding like the plot of a scary movie, an act of generosity towards a stranger, it's surprising that Paul didn't wonder if the driver had an ulterior motive.

His wife must have reeled when her husband arrived home with a Worzel Gummidge lookalike. Both husband and wife worked and she hadn't seen her other half for a few days because of his job. However, she was more than welcoming and showed Paul the bathroom, giving him some soap, shampoo and towels. This story made me wonder if this wasn't the first time her husband had brought a lost soul home. Paul said he had never seen bathwater turn so grey, practically mud-coloured. Before, he had been unshaven and filthy with matted long hair, and probably looked quite transformed when he emerged. He managed to down a welcome meal of lasagne and bread, even accepting seconds and a bit of cheesecake to round it off. He slept like a log in their spare room and felt like a new man the next morning. The couple provided him with breakfast and the driver explained that he had been able to make arrangements for Paul to meet the other driver who was heading to Scotland.

Paul told me that, although he had wanted to contact us all, when he had gone to bed he thought about his life in Germany and compared it to the UK. He wasn't sure how he'd be received in Scotland and was having second thoughts; he felt the time wasn't right to turn up on our doorstep. He had to explain to the man that he was sorry, but he couldn't carry on the journey with the second driver. He apologised and told him he'd given it lots of thought. He'd had a change of heart, he wanted to go back down to London and find a way to get over to Germany. The man was understanding about the new plan, cancelled the second driver and they both set off again towards London. When they arrived, Paul was handed £10 by this compassionate man who also gave him his address and told him to get in touch anytime.

A while later I put two and two together. I realised that when Paul had been in the north of England with the lorry driver, something strange had occurred. At that very time, I happened to be driving from the north of Scotland to my destination near the border. Paul and I were miles apart – he was in England and I was in Scotland – but we were both heading towards the border, almost towards each other. Nearly two years had passed since he'd walked out but, at a particular junction on the motorway, near to where Paul used to live in central Scotland, I had a prickly sensation in my body. Extremely strong emotional reactions and visions of Paul washed over me, I started to cry and then sob, so I had to pull over onto the hard shoulder.

I thought, *I wonder where Paul is? If I took one of these turnings I could try to find somebody who might have heard from him.*

I wondered what he might be doing at that moment, where he lived, if he had a girlfriend or even a wife. I smiled at the next idea, *Maybe he's a father now*.

Like Paul, I didn't know where to start. I didn't know if he was in the UK, Germany or some far-flung country, but in reality he was only a few miles from me. I didn't know if he'd be happy to find out that I was looking for him. I only knew his friends had previously lived nearby but I had no idea exactly where. I would need to have asked around shops and bars. All these thoughts whirled about my head until I realised that it was late at night and I had to focus on the road.

We weren't destined to meet again at that point in life but I remained optimistic that he might have turned a corner regarding his mental health. With more publicity around mental health issues and how people should be treated, I was content in the knowledge that if he sought help he would get it. During the rest of my journey, however, I had a few flashbacks tied in with regrets. Maybe if I'd done more as the mother of a small boy or become more involved in his teenage years I would have been able to visualise a different Paul.

And so, as I sat in the hospital with Paul in front of me, the lost years had been explained to a certain extent and I had the chance to help him build a new life. I could only do this by getting him out of Germany then bringing him back to what I hoped would be his permanent home and a fresh start.

Chapter 11

Coming Home

I had been reunited with my son; I couldn't let him harm himself again. Sure, I would rather our reunion hadn't been in a hospital in Göttingen, but now that the hurdle of removing the bullet had been overcome, I was sorting things out from my end. I was determined to get Paul back; I didn't want to leave him in Germany. However, some problems had to be resolved before we could go ahead.

A typical mother, my initial concern was that he had very few clothes, only the ones I had washed in the hotel bathroom. It was winter and I didn't want to imagine him coming directly out of a hospital environment to face the elements without a jacket or jumper. I contacted the British Legion, who agreed to step in and assist with what he needed in Germany and also to support him in getting back to Scotland. They sent a representative out to visit Paul in hospital a few times and told him if he wanted to pack up what he could from his flat, they would ship it over to my address in Scotland.

Initially, I had planned to get over to Germany a second time, not only to be there during his operation and counselling, but also so that we could travel back to

Scotland together. However, the medical staff's sudden decision to operate earlier than planned presented me with another concern. Paul's discharge was imminent and the doctors were letting him go without any counselling. Paul was upbeat about us finding a solution to his early discharge, more so than I was. Not only was I worried about his physical health after such a serious operation, but I was also concerned that he had tried to end his life just a few weeks before and I didn't know how to deal with this. It was a huge responsibility and, although I was delighted that the medical staff thought Paul was strong enough to leave hospital, I wasn't completely convinced.

Another concern was Paul's actual discharge from hospital. This weighed heavily on my mind, so I had to rely on Mark for a big favour at the other end. He agreed to take Paul back home to pick up paperwork and pack a box to hand in to the British Legion. Mark collected a wobbly Paul and took him to his flat. When they opened the door, they saw the devastation. He told me the carpet was covered in blood; it had been lifted and folded in a corner. The landlady had piled his few remaining belongings on a table and next to the sofa lay the stained towels and sheets he had used to stem the flow of blood.

Paul had discovered that the landlady wanted to see him regarding payment for the mess he had left, so he packed and sealed a standard-sized cardboard box for the British Legion and left as quickly as possible without seeing her. She never found him and, from his point of view, that was fortunate. They headed to Mark's flat.

The next problem was how to get Paul to Scotland. He could travel back alone, or I could go to Germany to meet him. The British Legion had kindly promised to pay for his travel from Germany to Scotland; however, I realised that it would be an extremely long journey. After some investigating, a flight didn't seem a viable option, whether we were together or not. Although there was an airport nearby in Hannover, there were no suitable flights to Scotland; the majority had two stopovers, France and England. The connecting flights between countries were hours apart and, all in all, the journey from Germany would have taken practically a whole day. I didn't want to risk him becoming frustrated and taking off again. Neither did I want a phone call to say he'd collapsed from exhaustion; I knew he had been signed off from the medical team, but they wouldn't have expected him to travel for so long and so soon after his operation. Although he was a young man, he wasn't exactly fit.

However, there was another option for getting him back home, one stage at a time. This possibility, although not ideal, seemed more attractive. Paul's discharge happened to coincide with a Christmas trip to Brussels that I had booked before I received the call about him being in hospital. Having turned fifty, I had wanted to experience a SAGA holiday; a chance to be with people in the same age group, or so I thought. A plan started to form in my head. I struck on the idea of including Paul, not so much for us to have a holiday, but to give him a chance to stop over and rest in an already booked hotel room a few hours away from Germany. Faced with a long, broken journey to Scotland or a short trip to Brussels, the latter seemed the lesser of the two evils. I decided to contact SAGA.

It wasn't an easy task to convince the tour organisers to include another person, and a much younger person at that, on the Brussels trip, but I was determined that he would join me, more determined than I could ever remember. I read their terms and conditions and it clearly stated that any member was free to bring a partner along, providing their place was paid for. I called and told them I wanted to bring a partner, a much younger partner, my son. Initially, I was told my idea was out of the question, but I argued that it wouldn't have been beyond the realms of possibility that people had relationships with much younger people, so I could have brought a partner who was the same age as my son. It shouldn't make any difference. Eventually, and they agreed.

The British Legion agreed to pay for Paul's journey from Hannover to Brussels. Although I was anxious at the thought of him travelling for five hours on a train, I could only hope and pray that he would be strong enough to withstand the travel. He had no choice but to travel alone on that leg of the journey. Then he would finally arrive for a few days' rest at the hotel, where I would be keeping a surreptitious eye on him. As far as I was concerned, the holiday, which I had been more than prepared to cancel, was now part of the overall plan. What was more important was that I would be there to meet and take responsibility for him. There was no chance we'd get health insurance given the suicide attempt, so he would be totally in my care. I had no idea what situation I would meet in Brussels and what I would have to deal with. But, as a mother, I wanted to make sure Paul would be protected in every way so that he had a chance to recover and I could then ease my grip little by little. At that moment I had to protect him; shield him from whatever might rain down on him.

On my way to Brussels, I was full of anticipation at the thought of meeting Paul in an everyday setting. Very briefly, I wondered if anything would go wrong and he might not turn up. However, I was sure he wouldn't step out of my life again and when my transfer bus from the ferry arrived at the hotel, I was delighted to see Paul waiting in the lobby. That was the first time I had seen him since the bullet had been removed and I could still hear his voice telling me that if anything went wrong: 'Switch it off.' But here he was, standing there as large as life and smiling. We would be able to celebrate Christmas together in a beautiful city. I really couldn't imagine how Paul felt when he saw the group of over 50s he would be holidaying with.

After checking in and finding our rooms, we finally had the chance to relax. This was the first time I had spoken to Paul in a normal environment for four years and he told me of his discharge, visit to the flat and travel to the train station. His yawns and narrowing eyes told me he needed to rest, to lie down, to relax, perchance to sleep. He had been through an ordeal and my excitement of wanting to talk to him at length would have to wait. Over the next few days, Paul slept on and off more than what would be considered normal.

At coffee breaks and lunches, he was the first to leave. The group joked about him leaving early because of the *oldies*: I didn't tell them it was because of his surgery and that, had he still been in hospital, the doctors, nurses and auxiliary staff would have been waiting on him hand and foot. He was absolutely and completely shattered.

Although he had plenty of rest at the hotel, I was conscious of his condition. Three days ago he had been discharged from hospital, six days before that he'd gone through brain surgery. It had only been twenty days since he'd been taken by helicopter to hospital and sixteen days ago my life had changed with the phone call from the Foreign Office. He was probably still reeling from seeing the devastation he had caused in his flat before he packed up and headed off to meet me. And here he was, with strangers, exhausted and with no idea of what his future held. It was probably all going too fast for both of us, but I didn't see that we had a choice. I was careful to keep my eye on his movements, his responses and his reactions. He was coming home, but to what I wasn't sure. I tried to put all these pressures on the back burner and enjoy the time I could with him.

There was one immediate issue we had to deal with; the operation had left Paul with a visible C-shaped scar at the side of his head. His hair had been shaved off, but only on one side. He had tried to disguise his wound with an old, faded skip cap. I told him I had alternatives, and produced a black woolly hat and, as a joke, a headscarf. Given the choice, he opted for the former, thankfully. He looked a bit like a cat burglar in his black hat, black polo neck and black jeans, but he seemed happy with his outfit.

It wasn't quite the city break I'd planned but I was certainly more than happy to forgo the organised group trips to enjoy short walks with Paul, discuss the future and laugh when we could. We both saw the funny side of the same things, which eased the tension of being in unfamiliar territory with people we didn't know.

On Christmas Day, the chef got things mixed up and dinner was considered a disaster for the elderly guests. Keeping in mind what Paul had just gone through, partly because of a lone packet of pasta, we were amazed when we saw the food being returned to the hotel kitchen. Unhappy guests stormed off to their rooms while we smiled at the men, who were tucking in no matter what was put in front of them. We watched the dining room empty bit by bit, then Paul looked at me. He whispered, 'There's a hospital in Germany where they serve blue nutritional drinks through drips! Free drinks!'

He was beginning to see how bizarre his life had turned out.

In Brussels, we meandered around Christmas markets and sampled the local food and drink. The trees in the city squares were covered in Christmas decorations. One had strange, blue, life-size sheep tied to its branches and at night, with the Christmas lights illuminating the square, the blue sheep were surprisingly attractive. Paul jokingly asked me if I thought they had been fed antifreeze, another indication that he recognised the strange notions he'd had.

At a market in the centre of Brussels, while people were milling around, a poor soul was making his presence known; the sorry-looking man was shouting at passers-by; generally ranting. It was plain to see he wasn't in his right mind. He was dishevelled, with long straggly hair, torn clothes and trousers falling to the point of embarrassment. His shoes were tattered and he was carrying a couple of plastic bags. It was difficult not to turn to look to see where the commotion was coming from. Paul saw him, then turned me around by my shoulders so that I was facing away from the man.

He begged me, 'Please don't look, Mum.' I'd already caught sight of the man but I reassured Paul by saying I wouldn't look. We continued walking.

Afterwards, when he told me more about his appearance and actions when he'd left Germany to look for our family in the UK, he could have been describing the poor soul at the market. The time he spent in the London area must have come flooding back to him at that moment in Brussels, and he wanted to keep the vision away from me.

We said goodbye to our SAGA companions; our short stay was over and reality beckoned. We were heading back to Scotland where there were appointments galore, first of all with the doctor, then a social worker, followed by all the services we needed to employ to ensure Paul could settle near me.

At the airport in Brussels, I looked at the departure board for our flight. Nothing was showing for Ryanair. That kind of situation makes me freeze momentarily. I asked at a desk about our flight, only to find out that we were at the wrong airport. We didn't need this. What we needed was a smooth transition. Fortunately, there was enough time to take a taxi to the other airport where thankfully our flight was displayed, and we were still on time… just. Heading through security to departures, I was a few steps in front of Paul when I heard the staff asking him to take off his black hat. I held back because I was sure this request was not going to be met with agreement.

I was right. It got a definite, 'No!' from Paul.

I stepped towards them and quietly addressed Paul. I told him I was sure it would be OK to tell them he'd recently had an operation. Reluctantly, he nodded. I said to security, 'If he was to lift the corner of the hat to show you his scar, would that be enough?'

It was and, breathing a sigh of relief, we went on our way.

We were finally winging our way back to Scotland, but our journey wasn't over. Although I had left my car at the airport parking to make life easier, we still had a three-hour drive in front of us. The December snow had covered the roads like a white blanket. Paul dozed on and off in the back seat and, while I knew a unique journey lay ahead, I looked at how far we had come with a sense of achievement. I crossed my fingers and hoped that I had arranged sufficient support for both of us.

Chapter 12

Settling Down

We stayed at my rented flat on the university campus the first night we arrived in Scotland. I had arranged for Paul to see the GP, Dr Lyons, and the social worker, Noel, the next day. I had made a point of meeting both of them when I returned from my week in Göttingen, to tell them of Paul's impending arrival and to let them know I was there to be of help to them as well as Paul. Now he would be on his own because I couldn't attend consultations or meetings between him and the professionals.

Despite his black hat, Paul presented well. Although he had lost a bit of weight, he didn't look ill. After his doctor's appointment, Paul told me the GP was intending to make a referral to the local psychiatric hospital, and he had also given him a follow-up appointment at the surgery. Things were starting well. Noel had told me he wanted to get to know what type of young man Paul was by talking to him privately.

As I had suspected, at the social-work department, I was asked to wait at reception while Paul and Noel went off into a side office. Nearly an hour passed before Noel called me in to join them. He said he could see Paul was a man whose personal care was good, with no evidence of drug-taking. Their private talk had revealed that Paul was now genuinely delighted to be near his family and he intended to make a life for himself by continuing to be around people who cared. Once we were out of the office and making our way downstairs, Paul told me that Noel had been open with him at the meeting. With straight-talking and a friendly demeanour, trust had already begun to build between them. We both came out of the building smiling because Noel had arranged somewhere for him to stay.

One of the rules linked to where I was living was that no guests were allowed to stay over, except under exceptional circumstances and even then only for a night. It was the same for lecturers as well as students. Living with me would have been out of the question. I had seen some of the desperate-looking people who came and went from the even more desperate-looking city hostels and I didn't know how Paul was going to cope if he was given a place in one of those. Noel had told us that he had a hostel in mind for Paul but it wasn't one I had passed before. So, armed with the address, we set off to find his new accommodation.

We made our way into the town centre and soon turned in the opposite direction from the hustle and bustle of the main road. We carried on down a street flanked by large, very old and well-appointed private houses. Each one had carved metal handrails leading up a few steps to oversized, wooden front doors. Most windows displayed colourful house plants and were framed by curtains with immaculate folds. The tree-lined street was quiet and, as we headed into the heart of this residential area, we spotted the hostel. It was only recognisable by its street number – a magnificent terraced building that had probably been a private residence many years ago. The reception staff were expecting Paul and, because the other clients were out and about, we were both taken to see his accommodation. I was told that was the only time I'd be allowed near Paul's room. The residents had access to their own small locked cupboard in the shared kitchen and, on future visits, I would be able to sit there and have a cup of tea with Paul.

Noel had given Paul £10 cash; apparently clients usually only get £5 but Noel had given him an extra £5. I never knew if it was out of his pocket, but it was greatly appreciated by the penniless Paul. After looking around his temporary home and agreeing to the strict rules about smoking, visitors and socialising, we took a trip to the supermarket. It was impossible to start from scratch with £10 so I bought some sugar, tea and milk for him and he got the rest. I could have provided him with food and money or even tried to find him permanent accommodation, but that wasn't the point. He needed to stand on his own two feet and I could see him swell with pride as he held his key; he now had a place to lay his head.

Paul was there for the next few weeks, except for during one exceptionally heavy snowfall that brought the city to a standstill. An important rule at the hostel was that if a client did not return at night, their room would be offered to some other desperate person from the waiting list. On his second day at the hostel, Paul had to leave for another appointment with Noel. I had arranged to collect him after the meeting to take him back to my flat for some food. As a treat after I picked him up, we decided to buy takeaway fish and chips. The relentless snow had started the evening before. Although the early-morning gritters and buses had created a passageway for cars, snow had continued to fall, leaving slush on the roads and a buildup of hard-packed snow on the pavements. Side roads hadn't yet been gritted and, as a result, we were forced to stay on the main roads rather than take the usual shortcuts. Paul nipped in to get the fish suppers while I waited and watched the snow falling. In the short while he'd been in the shop, traffic had started to build up and was now moving at a snail's pace. Driving was becoming treacherous. It took so long to get through the traffic lights and roundabouts that the smell of the fish suppers filling the car was too tempting for Paul. He had scoffed his by the time we got to my flat.

We'd spent so long on the road that the snow was lying probably more than a foot deep on the ground. I couldn't see how I could drive Paul back to the hostel. Eventually, after looking out the window for the last time, hoping that by some miracle the snow would suddenly clear, we realised we were in a predicament. Paul must get back to the hostel or he could lose his room. It was too far to walk without the proper weatherproof gear and the buses had stopped running because the roads were not passable. I didn't know how strict the hostel would be under these conditions, especially as Paul had only arrived a couple of days before, but I made a quick phone call to explain and appeal to them. Thankfully they understood, saying some of the staff had been stranded too. They allowed Paul to take shelter with me without blotting his copybook. We would have been back to square one if he'd lost his accommodation.

Before Paul's arrival, I had not only arranged to spend Christmas in Brussels, but I'd also planned to visit friends in the south of France and stay over New Year. I spoke to Noel and told him I was going to cancel my New Year holiday because Paul had another important appointment coming up with an army doctor and the date coincided with my trip. I wanted to make sure Paul made it to the meeting. However, Noel was not happy with me. He all but shouted an order at me, 'You are going on your holiday! Don't you dare cancel! You've got Paul started on a more positive journey – this will be a test to see if he can be responsible and keep the appointment without you. Don't even think about cancelling!'

So, after only a few days of helping to set him up, I had to leave Paul in the hands of strangers at the hostel. I gave him £10 as a New Year's present and headed off for a few days. Paul was never far from my thoughts. The amount of money I left him with might have seemed sparse and, at the time, it certainly felt like that to me. But there were reasons why I was reluctant to throw any more money in Paul's direction at that time. My experience had shown me that he was not only quite good at borrowing but also extremely good at forgetting to pay his debts. Maybe I was being overly cautious but I remembered his old ways.

Several years previously while I was living in the south of Scotland, I received a phone call from Paul. He was miles away in the north of England and told me he was stranded. He had managed to get himself from wherever he had been and was now finding it difficult to hitch a lift back to his father's house in Scotland. He gave me some information, which was new to me but quite useful. If someone is stranded, another person can call train ticket sales and buy a ticket, but it can only be a one-way ticket and it will be at a premium price as the booking is last-minute. At that time, I didn't know why he didn't have money, but, of course, I arranged for a ticket to be picked up at the station of his choice to get him back to his father's. Although I had bailed him out in an emergency, the price of the ticket was quickly forgotten, at least by Paul. It wasn't the kind of thing I was prepared to create bad feeling over, but it came to mind now and again.

There was another time when he was nearing the end of his army career and had come to Scotland on leave. He asked Cait and me to join him and his friends as he was throwing a party. She was making her own way down so I travelled alone by train and Paul met me at the station. I don't think we'd even left the platform before he launched into a story about how his army pay hadn't come through and he found himself short of money; he was wondering if I could lend him some. That wasn't a problem. We went straight to the bank where I withdrew £100. I had a lovely time, meeting his friends and staying over for a couple of nights. The loan was never mentioned and, yet again, I didn't see my money repaid.

I was pretty sure I wouldn't have been the only person he'd *borrowed* from and it was a habit that I didn't like to see forming. If this type of behaviour continued he would have become known as a sponger, if he wasn't already. I also figured that, with ready money, he could easily have hopped on a bus or a train and disappeared yet again. I considered if his having a limited amount of cash could perhaps curtail his movements, then that was a good option.

When I returned I learned he hadn't even gone out on Hogmanay, an extremely important event in Scotland. The residents and staff had planned to hit the party scene around 10 pm and invited him to join them. He remembered his £10 note and told them, 'No, thanks, I'm staying in.' He had thought to himself, *If I go out, I'll spend this with people I don't even know and I'll have nothing left, so I'm not going out.*

It seems the staff were annoyed because, even if there is only one client in the hostel, a member of staff has to be there on duty. Paul's decision was a good one, though. He stayed safe and waited patiently for a new year and a new direction. His decision to keep the £10 stood him in good stead for future choices he would have to make.

I was over the moon to learn that, while I was gone, he kept the appointment with the army doctor. It was extremely important. We desperately needed the doctor's opinion, not only on Paul's mental state but also to discover whether or not his problems stemmed from being incapacitated due to some experiences while he was serving his country. Depending on the outcome, Paul may have been entitled to a war pension as well as an army pension.

When we next met, Paul told me that he and the doctor had spoken for about ten minutes.

Finally, the doctor said, 'OK, I'll get this report off. You're dealing with some serious issues.'

Paul asked him how he could tell after such a short time. The doctor had announced, 'I could tell the minute you walked through the door!'

Although I hoped this meant he would be OK as far as pensions were concerned, in my naivety I didn't want to believe that there might be serious, lifelong, underlying mental health issues. In the meantime, we had to wait for the army doctor to write up and submit his report.

We had no idea how long Paul would be staying at the hostel and, although tenants came and went at an alarming rate, the staff took an interest in them. It was comforting to know that some local restaurants and cafés were aware of the plight of the young men and women, and I was told that often trays of food would appear from local establishments. Several times a week, I collected Paul and we went shopping or back to my flat for food where he would have a chance to watch TV uninterrupted. One day when I arrived to pick him up, I was in time to see an enormous tray of hot pies being delivered from a nearby bakery. The receptionist thanked the delivery man who set them on the hostel counter.

'Wow, that's a load of pies! They smell good,' I commented.

'Just watch,' he replied. 'They'll be gone in an instant.'

Sure enough, within a minute practically every door opened and the pies were demolished. What was interesting was that even though the tenants could have enjoyed two, if not three, they waited until everyone had had their share before getting tucked into the leftovers. Paul was lucky enough to get two and even luckier to have someone to feed him elsewhere.

After a few weeks of living in the hostel, a letter arrived giving details of an appointment with the council housing department. This department was rumoured to be quite daunting. No doubt there would be many who created problems and argued with staff as they demanded a house. Both the customers and staff must have got frustrated waiting for the slow wheels of local government to turn. Dealing with people who found it difficult to fill in the extensive forms, provide the relevant documentation and conduct themselves in an orderly manner would make these meetings awkward. As a result, Perspex partitions had been erected to separate customers and staff. Tension filled the air. At the main door, there was a security guard and another one who circulated to make sure everyone was behaving. There was not only a physical divide but also an atmosphere of *them and us*. I had suggested I could go with Paul as a support and he readily agreed.

As I was working at the university, I had to use my lunch break to accompany him. The black hat was staying on to hide his now healing elongated scar, and once again teamed up with his black polo neck sweater, the cat burglar look reemerged. His appearance could have been construed as menacing, yet inside he was shaking. Once his name was called, we entered a closed booth where a smartly dressed young lady was sitting on the other side of the Perspex screen. The divide was exacerbated by the depth of the desk she sat behind – we must have been about four feet away from her. I caught her snatching the briefest of glances at us as we entered, then she put her head back down and continued writing without acknowledging us. Immediately, I suspected this might not go well. She must have thought we were just another pair who would end up being escorted off the premises.

Thankfully, I had briefed Paul on what we might face in terms of waiting time before he got a house – the last thing I wanted was for him to think he was going to be handed a set of keys that day. Paul was watching my every move and I surreptitiously signalled to him that we would say nothing until she did. Not that he would have.

After what was definitely a minute too long, she looked up and said to no one in particular, 'Right, how can I help you?'

Paul was nervous but told her he was on the waiting list for a house. He hadn't given her enough information and her facial expression let me know she was, if she wasn't already, going to become easily exasperated. Her next question was answered with the same obvious reply. I felt he didn't have the social skills to deal with the questions or the situation. He told me later he was afraid to divulge too much. He didn't realise she already knew he had a room at the hostel and that this was a natural step in the process of housing allocation. I was heartened to hear that he was also trying to remain calm, which came across to me as not being able to answer the woman quickly enough – I had interpreted his demeanour in the wrong way.

I could see how these types of interviews would deteriorate into confrontation. I was happy to get involved where needed, and at one point when he couldn't remember a date, I leaned forward to tell her the day and month. My jacket opened slightly and my university staff badge became clearly visible. She saw it. Maybe it was a coincidence, but after that she appeared more friendly and explained the process behind being offered accommodation and suggested ideas, to the point where Paul became relaxed and was able to communicate. I was proud of him.

If and when he qualified for a council house, he would also qualify for housing benefit so he would have the security of knowing his rent was covered.

Chapter 13

A New Start

Paul was delighted when, soon after his meeting at the council offices, another letter arrived for him. He was being offered a first-floor, one-bedroomed, unfurnished flat with a private entrance at street level. He picked up the keys as quickly as possible and we headed round to inspect it. The good-sized living room and separate kitchen were more than adequate for one person. It was pleasantly located, complete with a little balcony that allowed him to survey the street and car park. He gladly accepted his new abode.

The Soldiers, Sailors, Airmen and Families Association (SSAFA) had given Paul food donations when he had first arrived and so I suggested we take a trip out to their headquarters to have a chat with them and let them know he now had his own flat. Initially, he had been scathing of the charity. It seemed there was a bit of a joke between the *lads* from the army when they heard of an ex-service person who needed the SSAFA's help. I could understand this to a certain extent, because when people are young and healthy, they can't ever imagine becoming older and ill. We talked about how he wasn't in a position now to jest or refuse, and he eventually agreed to come with me. Their office was on the outskirts of the city, so we made our visit part of a day out.

At the headquarters, we found a small group of people who kindly explained that their service was for anyone who had served their country and who needed more specialised support. From the leaflet I picked up, I saw they addressed the complex challenges ex-soldiers face: hidden wounds, depression, post-traumatic stress disorder, or low income. They are committed to helping service personnel overcome these issues and rebuild their lives. Paul was given another food parcel and some odds and ends for his flat. Then they helped us to apply to his regiment for white goods for the kitchen and carpets for the rest of the flat. I was amazed but delighted that they could do this for Paul. Their support and generosity made sure Paul would be able to continue on a new adventure, in which he could build a safe and secure environment without having to worry about how he would cook a meal or wash his clothes.

Paul started right away with the few pounds he had saved from his benefits, decorating the flat with bright yellow paintwork. This and the blue carpets funded by the SSAFA certainly gave it the personal touch. That cosy flat became his haven as generous work colleagues of mine produced items such as pots, tables and even a TV. My friend was selling a bed but it was too expensive for Paul, so I suggested I pay for half of it. He accepted and so little by little his flat started to become a home. He was able to put his stamp on the place, something that he hadn't been able to do for many a year.

I was just as surprised as Paul when his box arrived from Germany. The British Legion had kept their word and, although it had taken a couple of months to arrive, it seemed like Christmas again. He tore open the flaps, looked inside and stared.

'What is it? What's wrong?' I asked, unsure of what his answer might be.

He narrowed his eyes and laughed as he brought out a selection of tatty, cheap, well-worn items. The haul comprised, among other small items, a glass ashtray, two mugs and a book about motorbikes. He screwed up his brow as he took out a cushion with some kind of peace sign on it.

'What on earth made me think these things were of any value? Look at what it cost to send the box over here. What rubbish!' He chuckled as he shook his head.

I looked in the box and jokingly remarked, 'What? No pasta?'

Immediately I regretted having said that. He went silent. These were obvious reminders of how little he had had. Not so long ago, such things were part of his life. No doubt he could imagine them in his flat in Germany and I could sense waves of nostalgia; he now had part of Germany in Scotland. I welled up and turned away because I knew that there was a part of Paul that would always remain in the country he had grown to love; it tore at me to think that the pull might someday be strong enough to see him wing his way back there. I wasn't entirely surprised that, given the trauma he had been through, sadness rather than humour could creep in now and again. As it was, he was with me now and, until that changed, I intended to provide both mental and physical support. If he needed me, I'd be there.

It was only after Paul had been discharged from the army and was safely under his own roof that he could open up about some of his experiences on exercises and tours, especially in Bosnia. It took a while for him to get his stories out. Often it would take days or weeks as he remembered, bit by bit, the events that took place and how helpless he felt in delivering the aid that his job had demanded to safeguard those around him.

One day, I broached the subject of his role in Bosnia. I suspected the disquiet he displayed now and again could have its roots in deep-seated emotions from the theatre of war. I ventured, 'I know you keep in touch with some guys you served with, did you or do you ever speak about the things you experienced over there?'

'We didn't have time to talk about things; we flashed onto the next task and there were a few times we weren't always in the same unit.'

We spoke about how this might be a time to think about approaching the army and asking for, at the very least, an explanation about what happened but, more importantly, to point out that he was still affected. He said he had some stories to tell but that they might be difficult for me to understand. As Paul stood up and began to pace the floor, I asked if he would mind if I took some notes. He didn't, so he launched into a barrage of stories about situations that had practically destroyed him. He had set memories in motion and needed to offload them. He walked and talked, pausing now and again to light a cigarette or to look at me. I could only shake my head as I continued to write in bullet points. I tried to spell the names of the places in Bosnia he mentioned and the officers, who, he believed, had risked the lives of the soldiers.

As he strode back and forth, I listened, knowing it was important for him to share many of his troubling memories of army life. Eventually, I had to stop writing because he was going too fast for me to keep up, and to interrupt his train of thought might not have been the best move. After all, we could go back for the finer detail later on. I glanced between him and the paper I was holding the pen over.

Suddenly, the pacing stopped and he went quiet. I sat completely still, not knowing what to expect. In a split second, various thoughts ran through my mind. I wondered if the emotional strain had finally taken its toll and he couldn't reveal any more.

I was completely wrong. As he turned to face me I could see a glint in his eye, the hint of a smile on his lips, a relaxation of his shoulders and, as he breathed a sigh, he said, 'You know something, Mum? I feel great! I feel as if I've been able to get all the stuff out that's been going around in my head for years! I think I need another rollup!'

He lit his cigarette and continued to pour out more of what had been his demons. So there was light at the end of the tunnel. I felt privileged to watch his troubled past slowly melt away and promised I would try to make something of my scribbled notes.

I felt there might be scope to speak to someone about what answers, and maybe even compensation, he could be entitled to. I got the idea of making an appointment with a legal professional to discuss things. I went on my own to see a recommended solicitor and explained Paul's background to him, his previous disturbing behaviour in Germany and the medical input that was now required, in my mind, no doubt partly because of his experiences in the army. The process was that a QC from Edinburgh would be employed to look at the case.

Yet again, here were obstacles to overcome before we could move forward. Over four years had passed since Paul had left the army and three years was the statute of limitations to file a complaint. There was only one way that we could do this – if Paul presented himself as not being of sound mind to the solicitor, I could act on his behalf and we could circumvent the three-year limit. However, Paul had to visit the solicitor himself. I didn't know what I wanted to hear. On the one hand, if Paul was irrational with his answers, we could move forward with me at the helm. If Paul was having a good day and presented well, the solicitor couldn't take our request any further, and that could show that Paul was on the mend.

After their meeting, I went to see the solicitor again. He told me Paul had been able to conduct a normal conversation at their interview and there was nothing obvious to the solicitor that made him think Paul was unstable, so the case was closed due to the three-year cut-off point. Part of me took this as an indication that Paul was readjusting to what was going on in the world and I had to accept that there would be no claim and no possibility of financial compensation. That was countered by contentment in the knowledge that he might be able to move forward and put the disturbing memories from Bosnia behind him.

In the meantime, Paul was contacting family members and wanted to visit them. As I expected, not everyone was comfortable hearing of his return and that boiled down to them knowing he had been involved with a gun and their not knowing how to deal with someone who may well still have mental health issues. I appreciated visits would not be easy if there was fear or anxiety in the air, and there was enough of that from Paul. I remembered clearly what some people's reactions were and suggested we left some visits until later.

We started slowly, visiting people nearby and then venturing further afield. As usual, Paul donned his black hat and sat with it on irrespective of whose house we were in. Although it appeared rude, nobody seemed to mind or questioned him about it.

One of the first visits we made outside our comfort zone was to Erynn, a friend who lived in the south of Scotland. As a very young boy, Paul had been friendly with Erynn's son, Simon. Now the boys were grown-up and had made their way in life. Erynn chatted about old times, and it wasn't long before Paul relaxed in the presence of such a calm and caring person. At one point, I was aware of Paul taking his hat off and I held my breath. I hadn't seen this before and couldn't completely understand what was going on. We continued talking, reminiscing and laughing as the black hat lay on the sofa even when he went to use the toilet. Then I could whisper to Erynn, 'I can't believe he's taken his hat off! That's the first time he's ever done that in anyone's house.'

In my eyes, this was a turning point and I breathed a sigh of relief in the hope that a more confident Paul might be emerging.

Another visit he enjoyed was to his maternal grandmother and grandfather who had visited him in Woolwich during his basic training. He made his way down to Glasgow to see them by train – that in itself was a huge obstacle to overcome – and his grandfather picked him up at the station. He stayed overnight before I joined them. When I arrived I could see that the visit had gone well. They had spoken to Paul of times when he was a boy. His grandmother always enjoyed recalling the story of when we visited and he was in the bedroom being scolded by me. He had gone running into the living room shouting to her, 'Save me, save me!' Whether or not he could remember it, it always brought a smile to everyone's lips.

Paul's visit as an adult was very different. They had taken a drive and gone shopping to buy him a present, one of the normal things that he'd missed. He wasn't used to people buying things for him and, although he had experienced many acts of kindness from friends such as crashing on a sofa and sharing their breakfasts, he was affected by this display of being welcomed back. It was clear his grandmother and grandfather had seen through his present state of mind by remembering the *save me* incident and the young soldier who had affectionately hugged his grandmother on their surprise visit to Woolwich.

Back up north, we were returning to his flat from town one day. I could sense he was much stronger mentally than before so I broached the subject of his attempted suicide. I questioned him, 'Paul, it must have been a very difficult time in Germany and I want to ask you, do you think you would ever do that again?'

He insisted, 'No, I wouldn't.'

I asked, 'What makes things any different? If that was a way out for you before, why not in the future?'

He turned to me with a smile on his face. 'Because you're here now!'

That touched my heart but I thought, *What a responsibility*.

I spoke to him about his childhood and how I now realised that, when he was with me as a boy, I didn't always understand how to deal with life. I told him that, as a young single mum, most of my energy had been directed at the minutiae of life: watching every penny, hunting for bargains and keeping the house clean – things that now seemed quite unimportant. I admitted that, during his formative years, my focus should have been directed more at building up his character.

When I ran my concerns by him, he said, 'Mum, you've got nothing to reproach yourself for.'

I was astounded at his word usage – where on earth had he heard that expression and did he realise what he had just said? Maybe he had heard it somewhere before, perhaps in some form of therapy or counselling by Noel as Paul had tried to explain the guilt he felt about the situations in Bosnia. He certainly knew the context to use it in and I hoped he meant what he'd said. I got the impression that he realised why I wasn't always able to fulfil his childhood dreams.

With things falling into place with Paul, I was able to concentrate on myself more. My time in university accommodation had come to an end so I looked around for property to buy. It didn't take long to find a flat that suited and I didn't mind the ancient kitchen or bathroom, I had enough put aside to make sure the place could be completely renovated. The living room with its bay windows and the bedroom overlooking a grassy area didn't need much work but I was in the thick of it with the rest of the flat while jobs like rewiring, plumbing and repositioning a wall got underway. With gardens at the front and back, I knew I would have plenty to do for years. Laying decking, building stone walls and putting up a fence were in my plans, as was the idea of getting Paul to help with some of the work if he so wished; I kept that intention to myself.

Chapter 14

Financial Security

An important issue now that Paul was back in Scotland was how he was going to manage financially; social benefits were restrictive. The amount he was entitled to would not allow him to do much more than feed himself—buying clothes was out of the question. Applications were being processed—most had been successful and his social-security payments had started, but he had to be patient and wait for the army doctor's report. Although most parents want to help out where they can, it's not always possible to give financial support. That wasn't out of the question for me, but I figured it would be better to spend my time getting him back on his feet where he could become independent and support himself. For me to do this, Paul had to be completely honest with me about his financial situation. I could see he was receiving mail from a bank and a credit-card company and eventually he told me he had outstanding debts that had followed him. His social worker had asked him about this too, knowing that many of his struggling clients came with the baggage of having run-up debts. Noel had asked Paul how he intended to deal with this and Paul had said he would have to try to pay a bit at a time.

Paul let me read the letters and yes, the bank and the credit-card company were asking for large weekly sums plus an incredible amount of interest. Each month, he was looking at paying back more money than he had coming in. That was impossible. I asked him if he would trust me to deal with this. I couldn't promise anything – they wanted their money back and wouldn't be writing off the debt.

I called each one and explained who I was, what Paul's situation was and which agencies were involved with him. There was a fair bit of negotiating between us, but I told them that if they wanted any money back at all, they would have to alter the payments to a more realistic amount. In the end, we agreed his payments could be reduced to a fraction each month with not a penny of interest to be added on. His social worker was astonished, and Paul was delighted. The letters stopped and he could now manage his daily living with ease. He never faulted on the small monthly payments.

Additional benefits that he could apply for needed the go-ahead from his GP. Paul made an appointment with Dr Lyons and I wrote a letter for him to take explaining how Paul often appeared anxious and suspicious of others, making it unlikely that he could hold down a job for any length of time. Of course, the GP had all the details about the shooting in Germany, his visits to the psychiatrist and a report from the social-work department. When we met later that day, Paul told me that his GP read my letter and consulted his files. He had turned to Paul and said, 'Paul, do you realise you're never going to work again?'

I believe Paul had stared at him, not quite knowing where this was going, but realising this couldn't be anything other than positive. What the GP was essentially saying was that he was giving Paul the OK he needed to secure disability benefits. Paul walked home on that sunny day feeling elated. He said even his feet felt light; no need for him to go hungry again.

At that moment, neither of us gave much thought to how he would spend his time without working. On the face of it, Paul didn't have a problem taking things easy and pottering about in his flat, but there was no doubt eventually he'd have to be doing something constructive with his days. I kept the idea of evening classes or helping with my garden to myself.

We also felt optimistic when the army sent the pension application forms we had requested. Together we filled them in, giving dates and places and attaching the information supplied by the GP. I sent the forms and supporting evidence off to the relevant army departments and we were hopeful about what might come from Paul's interview with the army doctor some months before. I suggested Paul use my address as a postal address and he gave me permission to open any relevant letters. I reckoned that there might be a bit of negotiating still to come and thought it might all become a bit too stressful for Paul if he had to deal with it.

Eventually, letters arrived to say that Paul was entitled to two pensions: first, an army pension and second, a war pension. Also, the letters told that the army would backdate these pensions to when they received his application, but they didn't state an amount. We estimated he might get a few thousand pounds and hopefully two separate, regular monthly pensions. At least he was on the right track.

Shortly afterwards, a letter arrived at my house with a cheque for the backdated money from the army pension office. It was for a substantial amount, more than we had estimated. I spoke to Paul on the phone to ask if we could meet the following day, but I didn't tell him about the letter.

The next morning, as I was getting ready to go out, the postman arrived with yet another letter from the army and another cheque for double the first amount, this time from the war pension office. I couldn't wait to see Paul's reaction.

Once at his flat, I let him make a cup of tea for us then said, 'Oh, I forgot to say, a letter came from the army. You'll need to read it yourself.'

I slid the letter across to him, but before he had even finished reading, I wiggled the first cheque in front of him. He was smiling like crazy as he continued to read the letter, shaking his head in amazement. As he took a sip of tea, I rustled a couple of bits of paper.

I said, 'Oh, and guess what? There's another one!'

He jumped up to hug me with a cheque in each hand, knowing that this meant he was now to receive two substantial pensions on top of the allowances already awarded to him from the government. He was practically crying because these were no ordinary pensions he would receive – the monthly amounts were to be paid for the rest of his life no matter where he was or what his circumstances were. He had served his country and now he was being rewarded.

With his other benefits, his monthly income was taking him to a financial high he had never reached in his life and, of course, I reckoned the situation needed to be handled with care. I encouraged him to look back to the time I had given him £10 at New Year when he had kept the money rather than spending it. After a quick discussion, he decided he would seriously think about the best way to manage his money from now on. He could open a bank account and deposit the cheques. He was a happy, content young man.

While we were chatting one day, he spoke about the people who had helped him when he was practically on his knees and decided he would like to make a couple of small gestures. He sent his grandmother a lovely bunch of flowers and he remembered the truck driver and his wife who had been so kind years before. He had lost their phone number but he still had their address. There was no way of knowing if the couple still lived there, but I watched Paul carefully insert a £10 note and a short letter into an envelope then proudly set off to the postbox. It was probably a pointless exercise as he never heard from the driver again, despite having enclosed his address. Who knows, maybe some other desperate soul got the £10, but Paul's gesture was an encouragement to me. He was, to a certain extent, starting to pay back or say thanks to those who had helped him when he most needed it.

Now with some savings, he toyed with the idea of buying a car. Although he loved to drive, he realised very quickly that, depending on the choice, cars can cost an enormous amount of money. We spoke about people we knew and what cars they owned. A flashy car might give the impression of wealth to the gullible but these types of possessions came with a huge outlay, not only the payments for the car but the ongoing running costs, not to mention parking charges in our city. He certainly could have afforded a very nice car without depleting his savings by much, but he would be spending lots of money to have a car sit outside his door most of the time. He lived very close to the city centre and now had a free bus pass so he decided, at that moment, not to buy a car.

However, after considering his options over the next couple of months, he decided he wanted to have his own wheels and started looking around garages. One day he came back and announced he'd bought an old St John's ambulance with the wording on the outside painted over. He reckoned it would give him a hobby as well as a mode of transport. After paying the road tax and insurance, he started on his mission of kitting it out. He tore out the inside except for what would have been the narrow bed for patients to lie on, which he reckoned would double as a seat. Finally, it boasted such things as a fridge, a toilet and a small sink. One idea that came to him was if he resurrected the word *AMBULANCE* on the outside again and if he and some friends bought medical outfits, they could travel to T in the Park, a local music festival, and perhaps be allowed in free if they said they were there in an official capacity. I was sceptical, to say the least.

After he made a few long runs in it, he found the cost of fuel prohibitive; it didn't get many miles to the gallon. The ambulance didn't last long. He sold it for scrap and didn't, incidentally, make it to T in the Park.

BOOK THREE

Chapter 15

Making Mistakes

After a year back in Scotland, Paul was still having regular meetings with Dr Simons, his psychiatrist, Noel, his social worker and Dr Lyons, his GP. They had varying priorities: Dr Simons was trying to get to the bottom of why Paul had attempted suicide and what the voices had been about; Noel was concerned for Paul's social wellbeing; and the GP was keeping an eye on his physical health. Paul always kept his appointments and particularly looked forward to time with Noel.

Dr Simons thought Paul was, to a certain extent, displaying schizophrenic tendencies and eventually prescribed oral medication, but Paul hated taking it. Although there were no outward repercussions from the tablets, there were side effects, including feelings of discomfort and lethargy. When he mentioned this to Dr Simons, he was told that the choice was his; he couldn't be forced to take medication. I'm sure the doctor said much more, but that was the part of the conversation that Paul held on to and he stopped collecting his prescription. Not knowing the entire story, I must admit to being concerned about Dr Simons' lax approach to Paul. I felt he needed to assert his authority and lay things on the line. I wondered why he hadn't explained the consequences of Paul stopping his medication, but maybe he had, and that was part of the conversation Paul didn't want to hear. Appointments were becoming less frequent as each professional felt Paul was gradually leading a normal, safe and structured life and, therefore, no longer needed their constant input. Longer periods between his hospital appointments seemed to reveal nothing untoward showing up as far as Dr Simons or even Noel was concerned. I wasn't so sure.

At one point, I got word that Paul was to be completely dismissed from Dr Simons' psychiatric care. This was a concern because, although he was settling to a certain extent, there were still times when I witnessed tension and fear and, occasionally, some irrational behaviour. I felt I had to alert someone to what was going on.

For example, Paul and I sometimes went food shopping together; usually, he wanted to go as early as possible in the day when there were fewer people around. One morning, I could see him becoming edgy as soon as we entered the supermarket. Neither of us needed much, so we browsed a little. After five minutes, and with only two or three things in his basket, I saw Paul was casting nervous glances down each aisle we passed. I went to look in a freezer and the next thing I knew, he was at my side telling me he was going home – he handed me his basket and left without buying anything. There was no explanation about what had spooked him.

I was also hearing stories from Paul that added to my concern. Apparently, one afternoon, two women had glanced at him as they passed by on a busy city street; he claimed he could hear them talking long before they were even close. He couldn't tell me what they were saying, but he was convinced he was the subject of their conversation.

On another occasion, again in the centre of town during the day, a group of young men had walked past him. According to Paul, one of them laughed and said, 'Crackhead.' Paul immediately swung around and confronted the man who stepped back and denied even speaking, never mind addressing him. The men moved off but I wondered how quickly things could have escalated. Paul had to find a way to control his emotions but I wasn't sure how easy that would be if he was indeed hearing voices.

I wanted the professionals to listen, I wanted them to understand that I was the one seeing changes because I was in touch with him more often than they were. I feared that Paul might be on a slippery slope. So, to get the message across, I made an appointment to speak with Noel, who had also been informed that Paul was to be discharged by Dr Simons; he was just as stunned as me at the termination of Paul's treatment. We'd been through so much and come so far – I couldn't let this go cold, I had to keep blowing on the embers and so I felt it was time to tell a few tales out of school. I revealed that Paul was sure people were talking about him even when they were out of earshot. Concerned, Noel informed me he was going to contact the hospital. His reaction confirmed to me that Dr Simons may have been hasty in suggesting Paul didn't need further input so I made an appointment to speak with him myself.

Because of patient confidentiality, he couldn't tell me anything about what went on at the appointments with Paul but I could tell him what was concerning me. To begin with, I asked him what had made him think Paul was ready to be discharged from his care. He told me that although he had originally thought his diagnosis of schizophrenia was correct, he now didn't think there was anything mentally wrong with Paul, that he was playing a game; Paul's answers to his questions were 'textbook answers'. He suggested that Paul might have read a medical book at home and be primed and ready with the correct answers. This seemed highly unlikely to me. If Dr Simons had seen Paul's school reports and his spelling in the letters he had written to me, he'd surely have revised his ill-informed diagnosis. I doubted if Paul would have remembered the content never mind interpreted the theories of an academic psychiatric textbook.

I relayed the stories of Paul's deteriorating behaviour to Dr Simons, especially when Paul was in public places. I also told of another incident that concerned me. As we were driving to my flat, Paul became agitated, talking about conspiracies, political systems and how the powers that be can infiltrate normal lives and ruin them. He reckoned we wouldn't know which people were after us and we had to be ready to defend ourselves even if it meant *doing away* with someone. Guarding my side of the conversation, I told him that no matter what happened I would be there to support him.

He protested, 'But, Mum, I might have to take YOU out someday because you're part of the conspiracy.'

I knew by the tone of the conversation he wasn't speaking about taking me out for a cup of coffee! I told him that I would never harm him or be against him, that I'd always be honest with him and would never be involved in any conspiracy.

He countered my argument, 'That's the problem though, Mum, you wouldn't know you were part of it.'

I must admit, his threat had made me extremely wary. When we got to my flat about ten minutes later, I spoke to him about his 'take you out' remark.

He brushed off my comment with a quizzical look and scoffed, 'I never said that!'

That was worrying. After I had reiterated these events, Dr Simons agreed to allow a second opinion and suggested he contact a respected fellow psychiatrist, Dr Bell, who held surgeries now and again at our local hospital. An appointment was made, and when Paul met with Dr Bell, the result was staggering. After the appointment, Dr Bell called me and we spoke for nearly an hour. He was extremely informative and told me that he had diagnosed Paul with paranoid schizophrenia and he was in a bad way, hearing voices and becoming unnerved by normal life. Although he felt Paul would not likely be a danger to others, he had proved he could be a danger to himself if he felt his life was falling apart. I asked him about the voices, and if it was true that Paul was hearing them.

He categorically insisted, 'He hears them, he hears what they are telling him to do and he has already proved that he is capable of acting on their instructions.'

The conversation opened my eyes to the horror of what Paul was experiencing. I was deeply saddened that he was ill but also delighted that somebody had listened to me and now we could move forward. For a fleeting moment, I was so taken with Dr Bell that I doubted Dr Simons' credibility. I knew Dr Simons was a respected psychiatrist but there was no doubt in my mind that Dr Bell was more on the ball. I asked him if he would ever be able to deal with Paul again but he told me he would only be able to do that in conjunction with Dr Simons. He had the case notes and knew Paul's history. I felt I had to give the professionals their place.

I never kept anything from Paul so I told him what had been said. He appreciated that he would have to continue with psychiatric care, which was a successful outcome all round. The early diagnosis of schizophrenia seemed to tie in with his symptoms but, to me, post-traumatic stress from his time in the army would have made more sense. Perhaps I was in denial. His appointments with Dr Simons were to resume and his prescription was to be adjusted until he was happier with his medication.

In the meantime, and before any appointment came through, red flags went up again as he sat in his flat telling me that foreigners, especially Germans, were a real problem because they were likely monitoring him through the pixels on his TV and, once again, I realised I needed to take action. When I asked him to explain the pixels story, he went into great detail about how the aerial on the roof was acting as an antenna with two-way transmission. The discussion between us was quite lengthy as I asked more and more questions but finally, he shook his head and said, 'You don't understand, Mum.'

I didn't.

Early the next day, I went to the GP's surgery and asked for an emergency appointment for myself. I had to wait for an hour but I spoke to a locum doctor and told her about the foreigners and the pixels. I explained Paul had been more or less dismissed from psychiatric care, but he was waiting for appointments to resume. The locum said the only way she could take things further was if Paul was to come voluntarily to have an appointment with her. She couldn't do anything by taking my word as gospel. I wasn't sure how I could swing it, but I said I would try very hard to get him to the surgery as early as I could the following day.

The next morning, I arrived at his door unannounced and told him he needed to get ready quickly because we had to see a doctor. I said she was going to help and reminded him that the doctors were the ones who were the link between him and his benefits. I didn't give him time to think, even when I could see the hesitation in him. I kept repeating that this appointment would help him, hinting that the doctor was the one who controlled his benefits, which wasn't entirely true. I could see he wasn't happy with my request but he gave in. I drove him over to the surgery, where we waited for what seemed like an age. I prayed the doctor would call him soon because I could see he was becoming restless; he might have stood up and left. Finally, to my great relief, the receptionist called his name. When he came out of the consultation room, he said he had an emergency appointment to see Dr Simons the following day, but that the locum doctor had been questioning him about Germans. He was puzzled.

'What was all that about? She was asking me if I felt safe around foreigners. I didn't even have to tell her I'd lived in Germany. Germans coming to get me… I ask you!'

Paul explained that after they'd exchanged only a few words in her surgery, she'd made a call directly to the local psychiatric team. He could hear her say, 'I've got an extremely ill young man here, he needs attention now! His appointment must be set up for today or, at the latest, tomorrow.'

It was such a relief to know that someone had the presence of mind to act quickly.

Once I had deposited him at his flat, he said, 'Mum, I want you to make me a promise. Promise me you'll never do that to me again. Don't ever ask me to leave the house without giving me time to have a shower and get ready properly.'

I gave him my promise, which I kept. But then I had to press my lips together trying not to react at the cheek of him when he continued, 'Don't interfere in my life again. You just stick to what you're good at, writing letters!'

I didn't reply but I was inwardly laughing at his remark, unsure if it was an insult or a compliment. It didn't matter which; I had achieved what I set out to do and things were, once again, in the hands of the doctors. I felt I had done all I could to alert the medical profession that Paul still needed support. If things weren't taken seriously after this then I was at a complete loss as to how I could give them more to go on. I was spent.

Fortunately, appointments with everyone started up again. Over time, they tried Paul on a few different drugs until he got one that he felt was right. With his medication changed, his appointments brought closer together and Noel putting in some home visits, he was being cared for and monitored, but definitely not through his 19 inch TV set.

Now and again, he broke out of his routine as he became more confident in himself and tried to join various clubs, but these quickly evaporated into the ether; the childhood pattern resurrecting itself. He got comfort from religiously following certain TV programmes and liked shopping or meeting me for coffee. Twice he started short courses at a local college, English then psychology, but he didn't last more than two or three classes. During the first English class, the teacher had said it would be nice for the students to get to know one another a bit better. As an opener, she made the suggestion, 'Tell everyone about a near-death experience you've had.' Paul had sat there, his eyes fixed on the door, and asked himself if he should run. If he had opened up about making a gun and shooting himself, I think the whole college would have emptied, never mind the English class.

From the minute I saw him in hospital in Germany after the incident with the gun, I had tried to make things as lighthearted as possible and Paul seemed to appreciate the laughs given the circumstances. The college incident was a prime example. When he told me what had happened, we looked at each other, shook our heads and burst out laughing. An unbelievable situation.

Without the staying power needed for study and evidence of paranoia lurking in the background, it was hard for Paul to continue with courses and he was at a loose end. However, on one of these college courses, he met up with another young man, Andy. They would meet at Paul's flat and over coffees or beers they quickly built up a good friendship. They had something in common, Paul with schizophrenia and Andy with bipolar disorder. It seemed that the jokes and laughter between these two regarding their conditions kept their heads above water. Andy had a full-time job and eventually found a serious girlfriend, but he and Paul kept up their friendship. Paul had someone he could trust.

When he was able to socialise a bit more without becoming so anxious, Paul and I drove further north to visit Susie, a good friend of mine. Her children were very young; Cameron was only a few weeks old, a babe in arms. Of course, Susie knew about Paul's background and the fact that she worked in the field of mental health was a godsend. We chatted and the interaction was good. At one point, Susie was holding baby Cameron when she got up to make some tea and, as she was leaving the room, she thrust her baby into Paul's arms. 'Could you hold him just now while I put the kettle on?' she asked.

Without waiting for an answer, she was off. Before Paul knew it, he was holding the baby. I watched as his demeanour changed. He looked at the baby's face and smiled softly, even trying a few quietly spoken words to the tiny bundle.

Later I challenged Susie, 'I'm amazed that you trusted Paul enough to leave him with the baby.'

Quick as a flash, she qualified her actions. 'Who knows? He might never get another chance in life to hold a baby.'

Paul's integration into normal life that day became memorable and I looked forward to the possibility of the day when he would be holding another baby; maybe his own.

Chapter 16

Breaking Down

Paul was enjoying being part of family life. He was no longer the little boy who asked permission to say bad words or needed to check in before he went to see his friends. Although he'd had his issues, he was knowledgeable about things in life that I'd never come across; it was nice to be able to ask for his advice now and again.

I needed to buy another car, and Paul was more than delighted when I suggested we go looking around a couple of garages. Since he was small, cars had been one of his passions, so he did the research and convinced me that a Volkswagen was a good make. It wasn't long before we found a car we both liked. Paul did the test drive, gave the thumbs up and I settled on a second-hand, dark green Volkswagen Golf. I let Paul use the car now and again, although he never went far.

Shortly after I bought the car, my father, Paul's grandfather, passed away; we all attended the funeral service. I watched as Paul and the other pall-bearers took a chord and helped lower the coffin. I was sad that his grandfather would never see Paul making more of his life.

A few weeks after the service, Paul's grandmother was coming up from Glasgow to visit family immediately south of where we lived. She asked if Paul could come to visit too. I would be working, so I suggested he take my car rather than go by bus or train. He was thrilled and not only looking forward to seeing the family, but also driving the car. However, unforeseen circumstances caused the arrangement to be changed to a later date. When I gave Paul the details of the change, I could see not only the disappointment but also a dark, stunned look. It was as if I had delivered unbelievable, life-changing news. In my mind, it was only a car journey. For all I knew, Paul had perhaps thought he would fit something else into his journey and here I was, completely messing up his plans.

In the days that followed, I knew I wasn't seeing him or hearing from him as much. Four or five days had passed, which was unusual. After that, every time we met, he engineered it that we were at my house or in town. Something was amiss, but I couldn't quite put my finger on it. Then it clicked; I hadn't been to his flat. Alarm bells were ringing, so I called a couple of his friends. I explained I was becoming concerned about Paul and wondered what the friends thought. They both told me they'd noticed a bit of a change and one of them asked if I'd been to his flat recently. When I said I hadn't, he replied, 'If I were you, I'd get down there. I think you need to get inside. Don't let him stop you, you might have to insist, but you need to see what's happened.'

I had to tread carefully. Finally, I met Paul in town and once again assured him that, no matter what, I'd be there to help. I broached the subject of his flat and assured him we'd deal with whatever had happened. I didn't quite expect what was eventually revealed. Whether or not it was as a result of his trip in my car being cancelled, or some other incident that triggered him, but he had become raging and violent. He said his flat now looked very different and told me I wasn't to come down for a couple of days. He admitted that, in a frenzy, he had wrecked it. He'd taken the heads off of five golf clubs while demolishing his living room. The TV, coffee table and sofas were trashed. He told me he had battered furniture and walls to the extent that he could walk through the wall from the living room into the bedroom. He'd managed to preserve most of his bedroom and was able to use the kitchen and bathroom. I agreed not to go round until he had cleaned it up a bit and tried to repair what he could.

When I finally went in, I was astonished. His lovely flat was like a war zone, with practically nothing left intact. He was trying to get some semblance of order into it but all he had done was pile up the broken furniture. I was gutted. Things had certainly taken a turn for the worse and besides, I was becoming uncertain as to what the future might hold. I learned that Paul had planned for sudden getaways. He had two small overnight bags ready with essentials. They were both hidden in different places in his flat so he could lift at least one and run if he felt threatened.

Even though he repaired the walls and damaged doors himself, replaced most of his furniture and spent the next few months with his medication stabilised, I waited with a mixture of dread and hope to see what might happen next. Every time I heard the sound of emergency vehicles in the street, I tensed and yearned with all my heart that nothing untoward had taken place with Paul.

I knew I had enough energy to help him face the future if he was prepared to analyse what had caused his outburst and why it had been so violent. But it was difficult to storm in with questions and so I decided to leave it for a while and be of more practical help. Building up his flat, his confidence and reminding him that we were all working as a team to get on top of his mental health gave us both the encouragement to carry on.

About six months later, the unexpected piercing sound of my doorbell startled me. According to the two plain clothes detectives who stood on my doorstep, Paul was being questioned at the local police station. With a shake of my head, I indicated to the police that I wasn't entirely surprised; all I could hope was that it was something minor. However, in the comfort of the living room as the story began to unfold, my hopes began to fade.

It transpired that one of Paul's emails to a supplier of weapon parts had been intercepted and detectives told me that Paul was helping police with their enquiries as we spoke. He had tried to order a part that would help to build a gun. This was bad news for me but, initially, not entirely surprising as I tried to rationalise his actions. Paul certainly had a keen interest in weapons, considering the guns he had handled in the army, the gun he apparently had at Cait's house when he walked out at Christmas and the gun he had assembled to shoot himself, and these were only the ones I knew about. Once, while we'd browsed in a local hardware superstore, he told me that most people were probably unaware that from common items on sale, anyone with the knowledge could make a gun. I hoped he was joking. I didn't volunteer this information to the two detectives because I wanted to hear Paul's side of the story. They were now telling me that Paul was going to be released right there and then, but whether or not the police were completely finished with him was another story.

When a very angry and disillusioned Paul called me about an hour later, he spoke of leaving everything behind, heading off and completely disappearing. So this, it would seem, was exactly the type of situation that drove him to abandon all reason. Although I wanted to sit down and talk to him, I could tell by his conversation there was no value in pleading with him to stay; he needed to make his own choices. I begged him to sleep on it though, because often things look different in the morning. I told him if he did decide to leave, I would understand, but I asked him to please call me beforehand. In the pit of my stomach, I thought there was a very good chance that he would disappear out of my life again and I might not hear from him for years. I reminded him that I would be there for him and had to give in to the idea that what will be, will be.

I was delighted when the next morning he arrived on my doorstep and said, 'You were right, Mum. I'm not running away, we'll sort this out.'

We stayed at my house for most of the morning with me reminding him of what he had gone through in Germany, talking about how far he had come and how happy he was in his flat, well, except for the incident with five golf clubs. The appointments with his social worker and doctor were going well, his medication had been regulated and, providing things continued as they were he could go from strength to strength and have a fulfilled life in the city for as long as he wanted. Yet I could see that he was restless. When I asked him about the part he had tried to order he implied that the police were overreacting and reminded me of how he could have found parts in the hardware store. I wasn't convinced that he was taking this seriously enough but I had to let my questions go for that moment to get us onto a more positive train of thought.

Paul told me that the previous day he had been happy within himself as he set off to the supermarket. He felt a sense of freedom, which was short-lived when he was blocked, front and back, by four plain clothes policemen. Their demeanour didn't lie; they were people in authority. He froze as he realised there was no escape from the narrow lane where they had, according to him, cornered him. After they identified themselves, they pointed out another two plain clothes officers in a nearby car. They told Paul he could either take them up to his flat to answer some questions or go with them to the police station; they had some things to clear up with him regarding the email. Reluctantly, he had invited them in, where they disclosed that they were aware of his enquiry about placing an order for a gun part. They asked if he had any weapons in the flat, if he had used a gun before, what his interest was in the part he'd inquired about and what he intended to do with it. Given that the requested part had no other use other than to enable a weapon to fire, without question the police needed answers. Their concern would be not only for Paul but also for the general public. The part on its own would have been useless and so they needed to find out if he had collected more bits or if there was an almost assembled gun in the flat that was missing this final part. Paul answered their questions as best he could and explained that he had been in the Royal Artillery and knew about weapons and how to handle them safely. That didn't go down well. They asked if he had a gun licence, which he didn't, but, as he pointed out, neither did he have a gun.

Unfortunately for the police, they didn't have a search warrant, but they had heard enough to be concerned. In the end, they asked Paul to accompany them to the police station and questioned him further. They wanted to know why anyone would think about assembling a gun. He could only tell them he was interested in guns; he found their intricate parts intriguing. That did not convince the police this was a harmless hobby.

While at the police station, some things had convinced him the officers were being antagonistic with their questions and actions. He didn't think he had done anything wrong by emailing and claimed they had been provoking him so that they could arrest him. I got him to give me an example. They'd brought him a cup of tea but, as he took a sip, he realised the tea had salt in it rather than sugar. He suspected the normal reaction of anyone would be to spit it out with such force that it would splash onto the table, or worse, onto the officers. Then there would be trouble. He had quietly lifted the cup again and, in a very controlled way, let the salty tea run from his mouth back into the cup. One officer took the blame for the mistake, claiming the sugar in the canteen had been moved.

However, as Paul sat with me, he began to question things that had gone wrong in his life and rhymed off everyone he considered to have been against him, from close family to his superiors in the army. Exasperated, he asked me, 'Why does the system say I can't have a gun? It's not as if I'm going to shoot anyone.'

Just then, a group of laughing school children passed my window on their way home for lunch. I pointed to them.

'That's why,' I responded. 'Parents don't like it when there are weapons or violence around their children. We live in a country where most folk don't agree with guns because weapons can be a threat to the innocent if they fall into the wrong hands.'

He became agitated and demanded, 'Do you think I would shoot a child?'

I replied, 'I don't think so, Paul, but that's not the issue here. It's against the law to have a gun without a licence. As a nation, we're not comfortable with guns. Our police don't even carry guns unless they're specialist officers.'

He was blinkered; he couldn't see my point and he wanted a gun.

Eventually, I said, 'There's a solution, though. If you feel that owning a gun is so important, then you can have one. It won't be here, though. You could think about going to Afghanistan because that's a place where you could own a gun, probably more than one, and it wouldn't matter if it was legal or not. The only problem that I see is that quite a few people there will have guns and everyone will be in danger. If you're comfortable living in that kind of environment, then go for it.'

Unfortunately, the police weren't as happy with the email situation as Paul was. They felt there was more to this than met the eye and finally got a search warrant for his flat. Two days later, the officers were at my door again telling me that this time they had arrested Paul. There was no specific charge relating to an email requesting a part of a gun, so the only avenue open to them was to charge him with a breach of the peace. He would go to court in the morning, more than likely they would remand him in custody, and about a week later, he'd be back in front of the sheriff for sentencing once all the background reports were in. That devastated me. I asked them when I could see Paul and they told me, 'That's not possible at this stage.'

I interjected with a smile, 'Oh, yes. It will be possible!' I continued by politely suggesting that if they weren't able to make it happen, then maybe I could speak to their superior officer. One of them left the room for a few minutes with his mobile, then came back to tell me I had permission to visit Paul at the station. I put some toiletries and a hairbrush in a small bag for him and headed on down with the police.

They brought Paul up from the cells and, in the presence of the two officers, we had a short time together, maybe fifteen minutes. He looked quite stunned; he thought this had all been dealt with a couple of days before. He told me he wanted it to be over, and couldn't wait to get home the next day after court. Once the officers checked the contents of the bag I had brought, they allowed him the toiletries and then took him away. I put my elbows on the table and my head in my hands. Everything was out of my control now, but I knew I couldn't dissolve at that moment. My heart bled as I knew he was going to spend the night in a police cell. I continued speaking with the remaining officer. I had to find out what had taken place to create such chaos.

Once the second officer returned, I was told that, armed with a search warrant, the police had combed his flat, including the loft, where they found a decommissioned weapon, an AK-47. I had no idea what that was but I asked to see it. They stared at me in disbelief before looking at each other. I didn't hesitate and continued by telling them that if they wanted me to help, then I needed to see the kind of thing that Paul had received, possibly through the post. Although not on this occasion, he had used my address for some post so I felt I had to be educated in such things if I was going to prevent or at least alert them to anything suspicious in the future. One of them went off to investigate.

I had a flashback to a time not so long before when Paul had arrived at my house with a small, locked cash box. He asked if I could look after it for him. Before I could even ask what was in it, he informed me that it contained some personal papers and he wanted them in safekeeping. I couldn't understand why he felt his flat wasn't safe but that it was fine to leave them in my house, even though he had no idea who would be coming and going. As it was clear he didn't want to show me what was in the box, I was a bit hesitant.

Sensing this, he prompted me, 'Mum, you've got a cellar outside. Technically, it wouldn't be IN your house, it would be outside.'

I was pretty sure this was a situation to be handled with care. I felt there was something dodgy about it all and everything went through my mind – drugs, money, photographs – but I never thought about bullets or parts for a gun.

I agreed, 'By all means, you can leave it in the cellar, but remember the cellar in the back garden is part of my house. There's no *technically* about it!'

I could see he was quite happy; he thought he'd found somewhere for his box. He took the cellar key and the box was duly hidden. But by the time he came back in I had had time to think. 'There's one thing I have to say, Paul. I had a difficult life for years with very little money bringing you and Cait up, I also worked hard to get enough qualifications for the responsible job I now do. I work with children, I'm good at my job, I have built up a nice home here and because of all that I'm in a position where I can be a support to you. If I am found to have anything that's not legal or would give me a criminal record, I can say goodbye to my teaching career and my life will be over.' I waved my hand in the general direction of the back garden and the cellar, secretly hoping he would have an insight into his behaviour.

I continued, 'If there's anything in there that would cost me my reputation and my job, I'm going to ask you to rethink. Are the contents of the box so important that you might see my life ruined?'

He didn't say anything and we left it at that. He went home and left me with the suspicious box in the cellar.

I deliberated to myself, *Well, I'm going to have to find out, one way or the other, what's in the box.*

I slept on that thought and obviously so did he. Early the next day, he was at my door and right into the cellar. He removed the box. I never knew what it contained, but I'd learned a lesson – he could chance his arm but he had a conscience as well.

I was jolted back to the present at the police station when one of the officers brought in a long cardboard box. He laid it down then carefully opened the flaps. It contained the gun, which was in at least two parts, each looked pretty big to me. This was, apparently, the decommissioned AK-47. The sight of the rifle made my blood run cold; I didn't ask if I could hold it to gauge its weight, although part of me wanted to. It was a menacing-looking weapon for sure and that was without it being fitted together to full size. The detectives must have wondered at my state of mind as my emotional expression came out as a stifled, unhealthy laugh. I couldn't believe my eyes. All I could see was metal and a trigger. I knew nothing of the damage a weapon like that was capable of causing and I didn't want to know. For sure I hadn't seen a parcel that size and Paul had certainly concealed it well, not in the actual flat, but his loft. Although none of this was illegal, it was certainly disturbing. With a shake of my head, I indicated to the officers to wrap it up. My pale, tired, exasperated face must have portrayed what was going on inside.

One of the detectives kindly offered me a lift home and, once we arrived, we sat speaking in the car, specifically about what breaking the law in this way meant for young men. As I normally did, I told him I was there to help them as well as Paul. I followed this by telling him I wasn't going to be the type of parent who would insist my son was above the law. The detective gave me his number and told me to call him or his partner at the station if I needed them and they'd keep me up to date with any new developments. He said goodbye and I started to leave the car but, as I opened the door, I hesitated.

'Thanks for all you're doing, I know it's difficult because Paul's record doesn't look good and if he's broken the law, then he'll have to pay the price. Can I ask you one thing though – no more salt in his tea?'

He smiled and nodded.

Chapter 17

Breaking the Law

The next day, after a short, private court appearance that I wasn't allowed to attend, Paul wasn't released. He was, as had been explained to me previously, detained on remand to allow time for background reports. His destination was the local prison. I thought it would be a straightforward process to see him, but when I called the number I'd been given, I got the message that he didn't want anyone to visit. I practically had to plead with the staff to try to convince him to let me visit and later I got the all-clear. I was to arrive at 2 pm and could spend an hour with him. Only one visitor allowed at a time, or so I was told.

It wasn't an entirely pleasant experience. Strangely enough, I'd passed the prison many times without giving it a second glance. To me, it was an insignificant building until I realised that day what it was. Near a housing estate on the outskirts of town, one wall, visible from the main road, blended in with the stonework of surrounding buildings so well that it easily went unnoticed. The high walls, however, prevented passers-by from seeing inside and it could have been mistaken for a factory of some description. Even when I turned off the main road and into a side street, I saw the only giveaway sign: it wasn't a factory – *HM Prison* was displayed over the entrance.

A group of three young men and two women were milling around outside the entrance and as I approached, I had the feeling it wasn't the first time they had had anything to do with this building. I felt like the rookie, the new kid on the block. As I drew nearer, I could tell they knew one another. Passing cigarettes around, they sat on the steps, laughing and joking while they exchanged a comment or two with the policeman on duty at the door. These must have been familiar faces in this environment. I didn't know if this was a queue or maybe a group who hung out at the prison entrance now and again. Somehow I felt safe. If they challenged me, I was certainly in the right area to be rescued. The group never batted an eyelid as I weaved my way up the steps and through a mountain of discarded cigarette butts, a plastic bag and two cans of beer. Once I reached the policeman, he directed me to a small reception area nearby, where I had to give my name and who I was visiting. I was told to wait. I looked around at the four people who were already inside. They had got there in time to claim a seat, so I stood, waiting patiently. The voices from the group outside penetrated the silence inside and, if truth be told, their banter was uplifting. They recounted a story or two that would have made anyone laugh and I could understand their need for humour, their need for camaraderie, their need to escape the reality of whatever they were about to face.

'What's he in for this time?'

'Stole a bottle from Tesco. Third time he's been up this year.'

'Thought he was working. Why did he not pay for it? '

'He had a job with Willy the Washer, cleaning windows. But Willy sacked him because he took a week off. Said he was sick. Then Willy saw pictures of him in Benidorm.'

'What an idiot!'

'When Willy asked him about it, he said, "But I *was* sick, I just happened to be sick in Benidorm!" So that's him finished cleaning windows.'

Everyone inside smiled; the humour wasn't lost on us.

The group from outside came in as the policeman told us it was now 2 pm and time to move on through. I had never visited anyone in prison, but I had watched enough films to know that generally people can't touch or pass things to one another. However, I was surprised when a female voice from nowhere announced, 'Please use the lockers.'

I looked around to see who had spoken, but I was stopped from finding out more when a woman beside me smiled and asked, 'Is this your first time here?' I nodded. She explained handbags weren't allowed inside, so I followed her lead and used a locker.

They took six of us into a side room where a policeman told us to stand quietly in a straight line facing the back of the person in front. I was at the end. I almost fainted as another officer came through a door with a massive German Shepherd and asked if anyone was afraid of dogs. Terrified, I slowly raised my hand. He told me to stand still, not to look at the dog and not to speak to the dog. As if! We were instructed that if the dog stopped at any of us we were all to remain where we were and not to move away. The detection dog, or sniffer dog as it was known then, weaved its way in and out of the line and I held my breath. Even though I didn't look at it, I could sense the urgency and focus of the animal as it brushed past me. It never stopped at anyone so we were allowed to filter through to the next stage.

Inside the visiting room, the prisoners were already seated at tables with their backs to the walls and facing the centre while waiting for their visitors. I was initially taken aback at how everyone seemed to look the same. It took me a minute to recognise Paul as, like all the others, he was dressed in a striped prison jumper. He looked pale, tired and bewildered. No matter what the crime is, this must be one of the most difficult things for any parent to see: their child incarcerated and stripped of their individuality. Keeping a positive attitude while being completely ignorant of the system and how to act under these circumstances was a challenge. The chairs were somehow screwed to fixed tables which made it impossible to be ladylike. I clambered over the metal connections, dragging my legs through to clumsily plonk onto the plastic seat.

Strangely, my first thought was, *Why would they make everything secure? Why would they think anyone would want to steal these tables and chairs?* Much later, I realised a simple thing like a chair could be used as a weapon if an angry inmate attacked a visitor. I tried to instigate a conversation with Paul while looking out the corner of my eye at the mountain of a man positioned at the next table. I'm sure he could have ripped both chairs and tables up with one hand. I had hoped to get an idea of protocol from his visitor but, before long, the moment consumed us.

One officer was centred, perched high on a seat, a bit like a lifeguard at the swimming pool. Visitors sat with their backs to him and, from his position, he could easily survey the room. I put on a brave face and asked Paul how things were, for example, the food. He tried to make light of it, saying it was Michelin star and the service was like being on an aeroplane. He joked that a flight attendant came round with a trolley to ask what you wanted. He also made a few unnecessary remarks. Was I, his mother, meant to believe that staff would bring in a prostitute if he wanted one? He informed me he was sharing a cell with one other person and only able to mix with other remand prisoners at exercise time rather than with the long-term prisoners. He said that it was hard to get used to the screaming coming from other cells at night. The system trapped him and held his future in its hands. On my way home, I shivered at the thought of the detection dog and how the strictness of the day left me feeling like it was me who had broken the law.

A week later, they gave Paul a date for sentencing, but I was told he would appear in private again. I contacted the police after his court appearance; I had looked forward to seeing him back home and putting all this behind us to deal with his future. It shocked me to learn about the sheriff's decision. Paul wasn't released or taken back to the local prison. After hearing the case against Paul, the sheriff had sectioned him under the Mental Health Act, something I'd only heard of in media reports. He was to be transferred to Scotland's only maximum-security state mental hospital for the criminally insane. He was taken there that very day and I was given a number to call regarding visiting and contact details. It was brutal news.

Never in my wildest imagination did I think that such a sentence was possible for Paul. I called Noel, who said he had thought a section was a probability but had hoped we wouldn't have to face that. By now, everything was in the hands of the police, and Noel, Dr Simons and Dr Lyons were out of the picture. So, it seemed, was I.

I had no idea about the time limit of sections, however, I found out that initially, a section was for forty-eight or seventy-two hours, then a further seven days could be added, after which the section could be extended by whatever time the court felt was necessary. Paul was to be taken one hundred and sixty miles away from home and for an indefinite period. I was confused and didn't know what would happen next, but neither did he. I had to find out how I could see him again while he was locked up so far away.

The progress Paul had been making with the doctor, the social worker and the hospital had to be put on the back burner until this situation had been dealt with. Encouragement came from the fact that his incarceration was in an institution that specialises in not only those who have broken the law but also those who have significant mental health issues. I was now entering new and unknown territory, an area that was full of experts who could hopefully guide us in how to deal with the odd choices Paul had made and help me learn the correct way to support him.

And so it was that I found myself boarding that unappealing minibus and travelling south every second Sunday. This journey, its procedures, and my quirky fellow travellers, Bomber Jacket, Tracksuit and the smelly Kellys, were all to become quickly familiar. Every trip was similar, but now and again the driver made new stops and visitors I'd never seen before, boarded.

As the months went by, my feelings changed. No longer did I take in how others presented, but I somehow shared their despondency and mental exhaustion. If any of the regulars stopped visiting, I wondered why they were never seen again, but nobody talked about what might have become of them. Initially, I wondered if the visitor was ill or had allowed someone else from another area to go in their place. With a little hope in my heart, I imagined the patient had been released, then my hopes sank when I realised they might just have been transferred to another hospital. I dreaded to think that the visitor had had enough of the fortnightly commitment and had thrown in the towel.

Naturally, there was a procedure to follow when visiting the state hospital and, once there, every visit started in the same way: obtaining a photo ID badge, signing in and then joining the queue for airport-type security. Boxes and packets of goodies along with bottles of fizzy drinks were loaded onto the security belts as quickly as was humanly possible – everyone wanted through immediately. To the disappointment of several visitors already drained by their early morning start, the rules could change without warning. Lovingly made home baking could well be confiscated as a new rule now dictated only pre-wrapped packets of biscuits and cakes in their original sealed containers were permitted. Just as in prisons, mobile phones, drugs or items that could be construed as weapons were forbidden, but there were ingenious ways for contraband to be smuggled in and, as each new way was discovered, a new ban appeared. Bottle seals were tested to ensure they had not been broken and any personal paperwork for the patient was handed over to an officer. The stamps or seals on envelopes were checked for drugs and, if they passed inspection, they were returned during the visit. After security, in groups of no more than eight, we filed into a hospital minibus that circulated within the grounds. It took about ten or fifteen minutes to drop everyone off, so if a visitor missed the first departure they had to wait until the minibus returned to reception. Nobody wanted to lose fifteen minutes of visiting time.

The extensive, well-groomed hospital grounds were devoid of people. There was an eeriness hanging in the air. The relatively modern entrance to the hospital belied what lay inside: the wards. Some were built side by side, like detached bungalows in a housing estate, while others were randomly placed; many were old buildings on one level. There were separate male and female wards, spread out and accessed by a series of narrow roads and pavements. Anyone walking around was normally a member of staff or one of the security team. We would pull in a few yards from the ward entrance and, when a security officer signalled *OK* from the ward door, the lock of the minibus was released and the visitor let out. Keys jangled, locks clicked and doors slammed. A tangle of corridors led to the final door, which revealed Paul sitting alone at one of about ten tables.

Chapter 18

Another World

On my first visit, two weeks after his incarceration, apart from two women and a man who were seated far away from us, we were alone for a while until a few more visitors arrived. My fear of how I would find Paul was quickly overcome by the pleasure I felt at seeing him again. Unlike prison rules, we were able to hug each other. He felt thinner and looked gaunt; the dazed, shocked expression was still on his face. I fought back tears and the desire to tell him everything would be OK. Seeing me break down might have piled more guilt on him and he could have refused to see me again. Furthermore, I didn't know if everything *was* going to be OK. It wasn't OK at that moment for him and when I left, it still wouldn't be OK. I knew I had to find out how the wheels turned in such an establishment. But, in the meantime, the conversation had to be positive without inferring promises.

It had been almost three weeks since I had seen or spoken to Paul. He had been through so much without knowing what was happening on the outside. I told him I'd gone round to his house and double-checked that everything was secure. He reminded me that his electricity bills and council tax would be coming directly out of his bank account. The rent was paid automatically by social services, so it looked like we had the minutiae of life covered. Then it was down to the serious stuff. Where he was and how he got there.

He told me he knew something different was going to happen to him on the day of his sentencing. He was being brought up from the holding cells to appear before the sheriff when he overheard some officers talking about how they'd been asked to do overtime to drive a prisoner south. Somehow he had a feeling this was about him; his intuition was correct.

We knew nothing of the system, except that I would be able to visit the state hospital every second week. During my visits, the time alternated between passing slowly and passing quickly. He relaxed slightly during our hour together.

Windows on one side of the ward looked onto the hospital grounds. On the other side, the windows revealed an adjoining room that housed an oversized TV and a group of dazed and docile men sitting on sofas. I had been told that visits could last slightly more than an hour, or until the driver appeared to pick me up, and so I crossed my fingers and prayed that I would be first to be dropped off and last to be picked up. Every second counted.

After we said our goodbyes, Paul had to remain seated until I retraced my steps to the outside world. Accompanied by a guard who opened and locked the never-ending series of doors, I finally breathed fresh air. The large room where we'd met functioned as a smoking room, but not until all visitors had exited. Immediately we left, the men from the other room would swarm through and light up, not so dazed and docile now. Glancing back at the ward windows after my first visit, I saw a few faces smiling and hands waving at the departing visitors, but I never saw Paul.

On my next visit, I mentioned it and he whispered, 'Mum, I'm not standing at a window waving. I'd look like a crazy person beside them. They're all mad in here, you know.'

The irony was, I couldn't tell if he was joking or not. He didn't wave goodbye after my second visit, but on the third visit and thereafter, I would look back and see him watching me while he waved goodbye. He had succumbed.

During subsequent visits, we chatted about everyday things and I told him I'd been to his flat to check for mail and suchlike. Sometimes a few more patients would gather to await their visitors. Now and again, our attention snapped back to our immediate surroundings because of a raised voice or the sudden scrape of a chair on the floor, quickly brought to order when security appeared. We never looked round; everyone had anxiety and issues to deal with.

I don't know what I expected him to say about the daily routines within the ward, but he didn't sound bored with the showering, the meals or the rules regarding activities and bedtimes. Maybe he didn't want to worry me. I could have put money on the fact that, once he lay down at night, like me, he wished with all his heart he was somewhere else.

He discovered that, after four to six weeks in the admissions ward, he could transfer to another ward, allowing more freedom, but that would not be before another court appearance. In the meantime, this was his home. Nothing happens quickly in such a system. Eventually, after months, they moved him to a second ward, although there wasn't a great deal more freedom.

During one visit, I broached the subject of his father.

'Look, Paul, I know you haven't seen him for years but I wondered if you would like me to try to find him?' I asked.

He stiffened his body and looked into my eyes. 'No, I don't want him to know anything about me.'

I told him if he changed his mind I would do my best to locate him and see what could be done. It was left like that until a month down the line when he brought the subject up.

'Mum, I was thinking. Maybe you *could* contact my dad. I don't know if I want him to visit me here but you can tell him what's happened,' he announced.

Having thought things over, I got the notion that Paul was prepared to let bygones be bygones and see what could be salvaged from his past. I went through the Salvation Army, Yellow Pages online and other sources until I eventually got a telephone number for his father.

A woman answered. She understood exactly who I was and finally I was able to tell Paul's father what had gone on in his life from the moment he used the crowbar on the car all these years ago up to his present incarceration. It took almost an hour to cover ten years of Paul's life for his stunned father. I'm sure he would have welcomed an invitation to visit, but Paul wasn't ready for that.

Paul only had three regular visitors: me, Cait and her husband, John. Some family members sent messages, postcards and letters via us to him. If any formal letters arrived at his home address, I opened them and took them along with me on my next visit. However, on one occasion, I had picked up a personal letter from Germany at his flat, which I left sealed. When I got to security I handed everything over and the unopened letter created a bit of a stir. I was told they would have to keep it. As I was recounting the story to Paul, security came in and said no one could translate it from German and so they decided to hand the now opened letter over to Paul with a couple of questions: Who was it from? Why was it in German? The letter was from a girl he knew and they took his word that it was only a general chatty letter. He told me the next time anything came from Germany that I should open it – that way it wouldn't look as though there was anything to hide. He seemed pleased to read the letter; I had no idea what had been written or anything about the girl who had written it.

Only a few people asked if they could visit but I soon realised they associated the words *hospital visit* with times when they had visited a ward to welcome a new baby or popped in to see someone who had been admitted for a few days. Without question, the potential visitors suspected I was putting up barriers when I told them that, before they could even visit, they needed Paul's approval, plus the hospital would require a completed application form and photograph for an ID card. To most, that all became too much for a single visit. At one point I asked Paul if it would be OK if his grandmother visited.

He looked at me, practically in shock, and said, 'Mum, how can you ask that? Look at the people in here – she shouldn't see this kind of place. I want to see her but I can't just now. She wouldn't want to see me like this and I don't want to worry her. Please tell her, not just now.'

However, now and again I stayed over with her and kept her up to date with his progress. One of my stays coincided with a day I was scheduled to visit Paul. I had planned to travel from her house by public transport, but as she lived relatively nearby, she was very keen to drive me. Long before we set off on the forty-minute drive, I reminded her that she would not be able to see Paul, but I could tell the way her mind was working by her comments – she secretly thought the staff would never refuse an elderly lady a visit to her grandson. Her surprise was unmistakable when she saw we weren't dealing with smiling doctors and nurses sporting sterile white coats or blue uniforms, but keen-eyed security staff dressed in thick black attire more akin to prison wear. Sadly, she had no option but to sit in the sparse, cold atmosphere of the reception area, where the well-protected hospital staff paid her no attention from behind their reinforced Perspex barrier. I had asked them if there was any way she could at least get a cup of tea; they said they'd bring her one. I hadn't thought beforehand about suggesting she take a book because, unlike a standard waiting room, there wasn't even a magazine for her to read as she sat, bitterly disappointed, for well over an hour.

When I came out she said, 'I'm never doing that again; they didn't even bring the cup of tea they promised.'

I had made a grave error by allowing her to drive me to such a forbidding place then have her sit alone. Although it was clear to me that there was a very good reason why patients needed to give their consent regarding visitors, I felt her disappointment and wished Paul had realised she was a strong woman who could have coped with a side of life that was alien to her. I respected his request and explained as best I could to his grandmother that there might be a chance of a visit in the future.

During visits to the ward, an officer would circulate among the tables, keeping an eye on things and asking if anyone would like a cup of tea or coffee. This was a special treat for both visitor and patient, not so much the actual drink, but more so that we could share something normal and mundane. It brought an everyday habit into an otherwise bizarre situation. On one visit, Paul and I asked for coffee. As the officer approached us with a tray and handed me a plastic cup, I put my hand out to take it from him. Unfortunately, our hands collided, which meant hot coffee spilled over his hand and the tray. He was very controlled and, as I apologised profusely, he put the tray down on the table and left to get some ice for his hand.

I looked at Paul and said, 'I can't believe that happened. What a disaster. I hope everything will be OK.'

He replied, 'Well, we'll see after you've gone, won't we?'

The inference was that Paul thought he might have to suffer in some way for the accident. On my next visit, he told me nothing had come of it, but the situation made me realise he was resigned to every event having a negative outcome. Always on his guard, he couldn't or wouldn't trust many people, whether his suspicions were well-founded or not.

On one visit, I had a surprise for Paul, After almost begging, I had been sent the irreplaceable Red Book he had left at his father's. Having looked through its pages, it had surprised but delighted me to read that his military conduct had been described as 'Exemplary'. The security officer at the entrance looked at the book, then at me as I handed it over with other paperwork.

He enquired, 'Why on earth have you got a Red Book and why are you bringing it in here?'

I told him that Paul had been in the army and that he had left it behind when he moved house a few years before; Paul thought he had lost it forever. This was going to be a surprise for him, so I asked if they could conceal it between the other paperwork when they handed it to me in the ward.

He smiled and said, 'Of course! I was in the army, so I know exactly how important this is. I hadn't realised that Paul had served, I must have a chat with him sometime.'

Later, the officer came into the visiting room and knowingly smiled at me as he handed me the envelopes and paperwork along with the bag of chocolate and drinks I had brought. Most things were available in the hospital—sweets, crisps and cakes—but it seemed rude to appear empty-handed and so patients welcomed the stack of goodies that spilled out of plastic bags. Paul rifled through his bag then, after dealing with other papers, I slipped my hand under a large brown envelope and felt for the Red Book. As I pulled it out I watched his face.

'Where the hell did you get that?' he asked with a look of complete amazement.

I told him that I'd managed to contact his father, who had sent it on to me. Paul kept slowly shaking his head. At the end of the visit, he asked me to keep it safe at home: he had his irreplaceable treasure back.

I learned that, once a year, the state hospital hosted an open day where visitors and patients could mingle in the hospital grounds outwith normal visiting hours. Unfortunately, I couldn't attend because of unavoidable work commitments. On my next visit following the open day, Paul told me there had been stalls, drinks and snacks, and the patients had the freedom to move around with any friends or family who had managed to visit. He said he had looked for me all day, despite the fact I'd told him I couldn't make it. I sensed I'd let him down, and once again felt the added pressure of him being so far away from home. But, he had enjoyed the open day. He had quietly milled around for a while but then had become quite animated when he saw a shooting range. He had thought, *This is the stall for me*. He made straight for it, was given a gun, fired a few dummy bullets and won a holdall. Nobody seemed to bat an eyelid. I guess if the stall owner had been warned that Paul purported to be a crack shot he might have shut up shop early for fear of losing all his prizes.

It seemed that, now and again, the patients would have a bit of a lighthearted laugh at the expense of each other, or of the staff. Paul told me about one patient who had a regular appointment with a female hospital psychiatrist. Paul knew who she was but he wasn't under her care. He described her as being in her early 30s, medium height, not exactly slim, with long hair and always wearing a large pair of dark-rimmed glasses. Armed with a clipboard she took the patient off for, in Paul's opinion, a very short interview. Back in the ward, half a dozen or so patients sat on the sofas waiting for some comment from the patient.

'Well,' he announced, 'that was a waste of good smoking time.'

They acknowledged his feelings by nodding.

'In the end, she asked me if there was anything I wanted to add.'

The others craned their necks in anticipation.

'I leaned forward and looked right into her eyes one at a time and told her, "Aye, you should have gone to Specsavers!" Clever, eh?'

However, despite joking around, Paul hated the situation. He knew he had no cause to complain because he had broken the law, and didn't expect to be locked up in five-star accommodation. Most patients, and sometimes staff, made life uncomfortable for him; the showers were one of his pet hates. In general, the men were brutal in their talk and brutal in their actions. The only way Paul could be comfortable was to make sure he was up early enough to be first in and first out of the showers. It happened occasionally that he wasn't let out of his room until the showers were full. But he didn't complain.

On one occasion, he passed the staff desk and saw a pair of earphones lying there; he realised they were exactly like one of two sets he had in his locker. When he went to get his, one set was gone. Maybe they had fallen out and nobody knew where they had come from, but he was fearful of questioning anyone in authority about it, something that he had learned not to do in the army. He told me the staff did spot checks of lockers every so often and he was sure they just took what they wanted; he said no more, but part of me wondered if he really had a second set or if he was imagining the whole situation.

I learned that part of the problem in dealing with serious mental health issues is not knowing what to believe.

Paul told me the nature of some of his fellow patients' crimes. One young man had murdered his friend during a dispute over a game of cards. Another had killed his brother as they worked on a farm together. Paul's crime didn't seem on a par with theirs, but he had broken the law and the court had decided he had to be in with murderers and every other kind of serious offender. Guns, knives and deadly weapons would have been commonplace in their lives; not much different from Paul's life it seemed. And so he found himself surrounded by hardened, criminally insane men whose rap sheets made Paul's breach of peace charge seem like child's play.

Occasionally, on the return bus journey when the atmosphere was slightly more relaxed, people sometimes shared their stories. Two sisters who always travelled together told me that, as a teenager, their older sister had lashed out at their mother. The sister had been causing a few problems at home and this was the last straw. Their father had agreed to have her sectioned and she had been in mental institutions ever since. She had spent nearly thirty years of her life locked away with no release date. I asked if they'd spoken to the medical team to see what could be done.

One sister told me, 'No, we never bothered. We wouldn't know what to say to them and they're in charge. Now there's no one to look after her on the outside so she's just as well being in here.'

There was another older couple who told me their son had been in the state hospital for over ten years because he had severely disfigured another man in a fight. Although there was no fixed term for patients, I learned that the average stay was around twenty years. Suddenly I became miserable. Surely that couldn't possibly be the case with Paul? He'd already been in for almost a year. I couldn't leave him there without helping him to fight his corner. He had broken the law and maybe he would never get out, but the medical profession needed to know that I would try very hard to be the support he needed if he was at least nearer home. My hopes diminished the more I heard about the background of some of the men and women who had become institutionalised.

For a while it was like I had fallen from a capsized boat, struggling, out of my depth and without a rescuer. On one hand, Paul could be detained indefinitely, but on the other hand if I could fight his corner, there was more hope of him being released than if he had been placed in prison with a definitive sentence. If that had happened, I wouldn't have had the chance to put forward a case for having Paul moved nearer to home.

Rather than spend hours on the bus every second Sunday doing nothing much, I flitted between reading a book or picking up some task for a postgraduate degree course I had enrolled in. By the time the weeks had turned into months, I had managed to complete many an assignment towards my course on that bus. I didn't enjoy sitting silently mulling over negative thoughts on my way to visit Paul; there was time enough for that after my visits.

Once visiting was over and we boarded our bus again, unless specifically requested, there were no comfort breaks on the return journey, which meant three hours travelling before the first passenger was dropped off. The mood was slightly different and we dared to breathe a sigh of relief. It was usually dark when the visitors touched familiar ground in the cold night air. Back home, I could kick off my shoes in the comfort of my own home and let my feelings run riot. There was no such freedom for Paul, and after each visit, I was left with the same unanswered question: When will this end?

BOOK FOUR

Chapter 19

Nearer Home

I was at a loss as to what I could do to infiltrate the workings of the system in the state hospital without appearing rude or overbearing. In the early days, my energy was at a low ebb and it took me all my time to plan around visits to Paul. I had to get back on track before I could think about who to contact and who could help. I had always made sure there was good communication between myself and the staff and, as the months passed, my determination started to resurface.

I found a contact in our local psychiatric hospital in the north, a Dr Barrie. Paul's original psychiatrist, Dr Simons, had had to pass the case on after the arrest. Now that I had a name, I made an appointment. I didn't mention anything to Paul because I had no idea where it would lead. At our first meeting, Dr Barrie told me that he was the main link between the state hospital and the north. He decided who stayed, who moved, and to a certain extent, who was released. We discussed where Paul had been placed and he conceded that probably placing him in such a secure setting was not fully justified. After reading the background reports, the legal team had concluded that Paul might pose a risk if he were placed in a less secure institution. Because he had been army-trained, the authorities believed it wouldn't be long before he devised a plan to escape. That had never entered my mind, but I don't know if it was something he had thought about or was even capable of doing.

By the time Paul had been in the state hospital for ten months, we all wanted this to end. I was convinced that, with increased influence and unwavering support from immediate family and friends, Paul would slowly begin to think rationally. Dr Barrie told me he visited the state hospital more or less every two months, mainly when he had a few people to assess. I asked him if it were at all possible, given his busy schedule, for him to at least talk with Paul. If he could give me his professional opinion whether or not there was a chance of Paul ever being moved out of the state hospital, then I would know where I stood. He assured me he would pencil in a meeting but said his next visit wouldn't be until a few weeks hence.

I waited patiently and, following Dr Barrie's visit and appointment with Paul, arranged another meeting with him. He said that having Paul up north was not out of the question. He had put some suggestions to the staff – one proposal was to hold a case conference, which I could request to attend. This was an opportunity for everyone to have their say regarding Paul's welfare after almost a year in hospital. To my delight, my attendance request was granted, but the meeting was to take place on a weekday. Because the hospital was situated in such a remote area and very difficult to get to by public transport, I went down the night before and stayed in a bed and breakfast. In the morning, I ordered a taxi. I told the driver where I was going and he remarked that the hospital was a terrible place.

'It's unbelievable how many crazy people are in there. I don't envy your job,' he remarked. He must have thought I was part of a medical team. I managed to make a sound that was neither an agreement nor a disagreement and never uttered a word about going to participate in my son's case conference.

The well-proportioned conference room door opened to reveal an array of seats which formed a circle. People filtered in. As well as Paul and I, among the group were psychiatrists, doctors, duty staff and an appointed advocate. Over the next hour, each presented a résumé of how they felt Paul was coping and what their recommendations for the next steps were. The main point of discussion was that Paul did not want to take the medication they were offering. At various points, they asked him to respond and if he had any questions. How was he coping in a different ward? Did he have any complaints? How did he feel about his actions in the past? Did he understand why he was where he was?

I watched Paul practically fighting for his life at this conference, and I knew he was at the mercy of the system. It pleasantly surprised me he could communicate rationally. I had expected him to pass a smart remark or two, but he didn't. Everyone, including the medical team, wanted to see him back near his family, but ultimately, Paul had to mull over what his options were. After the conference, he and I sat with his advocate and another member of staff. The staff member laid it on the line for Paul. She said, 'You want to go back up north?'

Paul nodded, 'Of course. I don't see why I can't.'

She continued, 'Well, the truth is you won't be able to go anywhere until you agree to take the medication. They won't even start to consider you for a transfer.'

That was the choice. No medication and be locked up indefinitely, or agree to try medication and the application to transfer to a medium security hospital where I lived would be considered. Paul agreed to try medication. Although to a certain extent, he had been put in a corner, I was relieved at his decision. My hands would have been tied if he'd stayed there, whereas in the north, we could, hopefully, work towards a release date and see him back in his flat once again.

And so the weeks went by. I continued to visit every second Sunday and watched him develop a little pot belly, one of the side effects of the medication. He was given short, escorted trips outside: a chance for a walk with two officers in the countryside and then a trip to a local loch. These excursions were aimed at building up trust and communication between Paul and the staff; thankfully he hadn't created a problem or tried to escape.

There was one special trip he made, much longer than the others. Given that his grandmother had been sorely disappointed at not being allowed to visit him almost a year beforehand, I saw a chance for grandmother and grandson to be reunited and for stronger connections to be made with the family. The social worker and staff at the hospital listened to my request regarding Paul visiting me. His grandmother was approaching eighty and was spending her birthday with us. I put it to them that, given her age, it might have been one of the last major birthdays he could share with her.

My application was considered. A state hospital social worker, Robin, came up north to meet with Cait and me a couple of weeks before the birthday visit was to take place. He checked the layout of my house, asked me about window access, routes in and out, and inspected the outside garden area for the height of walls and gates. He wanted to know about the other family members who would be joining the get-together. After consultation between the professionals and the social worker, it was agreed that Paul could be brought up for a few hours. I had been told there would be three people accompanying him and I'd also invited his social worker, Noel, to join us later. I never told Paul's grandmother what was happening.

We stifled a laugh when, on seeing the buffet, she commented, 'It looks like there's enough food here to feed an army!'

The minute I saw the car draw up at my house, I stepped outside without her knowledge and introduced myself to the officers who were, thankfully, dressed in casual clothes. I asked if they would please allow Paul to walk into the living room by himself. Outside, I pointed through the window to where his grandmother sat facing away from the window, unaware of her surprise guests. They already knew that, apart from the door, the window was the only escape route from the front. They let him go in alone.

Turning around to look at who was coming in, she breathed in sharply. 'Paul!' she squealed as she jumped up. She hugged him, took a step back to look at him from top to toe, hugged him again and kept repeating, 'Paul, Paul, oh Paul, Paul!'

Finally, he said, 'OK, OK, that's my name, Nana!'

We all burst out laughing, then she took a perfectly ironed handkerchief out to wipe her tears away. She probably got a bigger surprise when three others followed him in. However, because they weren't in uniform, I could introduce them as the people who had driven Paul up from the hospital; they wished her Happy Birthday. We took pictures while Paul stood in front of his grandmother holding a birthday cake, waiting for her to blow out the candles. He appeared quite different in this new environment; however, his dark blue tracksuit and strange hairstyle contrasted starkly with his neatly turned-out grandmother.

She looked at him quizzically. 'Paul, what have you done with your hair? Is that a ponytail?'

'Yeah, it's my new style. Do you like it?'

She leaned forward to get a better look and shook her head. 'Not really, it makes you look like a lassie!'

He laughed at her expression. The banter went on and everyone tucked into the spread in front of them. We had a lovely day. Noel arrived with a huge birthday bouquet for Paul's grandmother and we chatted about things that had changed. I showed Paul my new mobile phone, but he was completely out of touch with how it might work. In the time he'd been away, he didn't have access to technology, and I realised those who had been locked away for twenty or thirty years would be lost in the outside world. I put these thoughts aside and focused on the day at hand.

With the buffet practically demolished, Paul and Noel took the chance to speak privately in another room. Throughout the visit, the officers were extremely discreet in making sure they had Paul in their sight at all times. One officer offered to help with the washing-up; she surreptitiously covered an exit. We chatted while we tidied up and she told me that, on the three-hour journey up north, Paul had pointed out various places where he had lived; she could see he was enjoying reminiscing about his childhood and how much he was looking forward to seeing his family, even if it was only for a short while.

After a few hours, the officers told us we had about half an hour left before we would have to say goodbye to Paul. They gave him some time alone with his grandmother before leaving on their journey back. Paul had proved he was not intending to run and, hopefully, there would be a glowing report about his conduct on his day out.

Dr Barrie scheduled his next visit several weeks after his first meeting with Paul. Once again, I met with him beforehand to find out what he would look for this time. We spoke positively about Paul's trips out and his behaviour inside. However, Dr Barrie was not only hoping that Paul had continued with the medication but also that he was having some insight into his condition. I pinned him down to a date when he would visit and I told him I'd like to see him in the office the day after.

He said in a friendly, knowing voice, 'Oh, I thought you would!'

His visit to Paul went ahead and I did as I'd said – I kept my appointment the next day and Cait came with me. The minute I walked into Dr Barrie's office, I hoped I was right in thinking I detected a little smile on his face. The clouds cleared, the stars shone and my heavy heart lifted that day. Paul had come to realise there had been something wrong with his mental state and he wanted to change that. He appreciated that trying to make a gun wasn't acceptable behaviour and, if he wanted to be part of society, he had to abide by the rules. He was continuing to take his medication and there was no mention of hearing any more voices or people talking to him through the television. He had conducted himself impeccably on his escorted visits and he had shown he could act rationally for a sustained period. I was able to get dates and times from Dr Barrie and the way the transfer would take place. After fifteen months, Paul was to be brought up first thing the following Thursday morning and admitted to the local hospital. I was so excited I had to let Paul know.

The procedure in the state hospital was that to speak to a patient by phone, the caller had to talk to ward staff first. Then they organised for the patient to call back but only for a limited time, for as long as one 10p coin allowed. On a Tuesday I called the ward and asked them how Paul was, before telling them I had spoken to Dr Barrie and knew Paul was being transferred. They also knew the relocation was happening but, as they didn't have all the signed paperwork in front of them, they hadn't told Paul. The transfer was imminent and I'd had the information straight from the horse's mouth, so I told them I'd like to let Paul know during the phone call. I was given the go-ahead.

Five minutes later, when he called with his 10p, I asked him what he'd been doing that day and what he'd be doing the following day. Then I said, 'So, what are you doing on Thursday, Thursday morning I mean?'

'What? I don't know, maybe playing football.'

'No, you're not. You're coming back up here.'

He yelled, 'What? What are you saying? Wait, Mum, someone's come in with a 20p for me.' I heard the money going in then, 'What are you talking about?'

I proceeded to tell him about my meetings with Dr Barrie and how pleased he had been with Paul's progress. I continued telling him he'd be coming up by car to the local hospital but that I wouldn't be allowed to visit for a couple of weeks. He gave some short laughs, I guess because he was lost for words.

Finally, he asked, 'How on earth did you manage that?'

I replied jokingly, 'Because I'm a wonderful mother!'

Although I had come to know Dr Barrie, I wasn't familiar with the hospital. It didn't have a normal wards or accident and emergency; it was a hospital for those with mental health issues. I had never visited the hospital or the facilities offered; neither did I ask to see them. I only knew there were locked wards, outpatient, inpatient and day-care areas. The main point for me was that Paul would be nearer home and I would be able to see him more often.

Later that day, all the paperwork was in place and wheels were put in motion. However, Paul was still suspicious of everyone and carved out a simple plan to ensure everything went smoothly for his transfer to go ahead.

In the state hospital, at the end of each day, there were two evening slots, 6 pm and 9 pm, where patients were able to go into their rooms for the night; their doors would be locked and not opened again until the morning. Most patients waited until 9 pm, choosing to watch TV or chat. The night before he was due to depart, Paul made a decision – he would take the 6 pm slot. He told me later that he decided to go early because he couldn't risk anyone finding out he was leaving the next morning. They might have become angry and deemed his *good luck* to be unfair. He said a fight could have broken out and, if he was in any way involved, he wouldn't be going anywhere.

The plan went ahead, and on Thursday morning after breakfast, staff took Paul to a waiting car and, along with two officers, he was driven out of the state mental hospital forever. I waited patiently until I could visit him in his new abode. We were now breaking the back of his mental health issues and none of us wanted to see that place again.

Chapter 20

Near Normality

Ten days later, I saw a contented Paul in his new surroundings. The first few months in the local hospital were not much different from the state hospital, except that he could have more visits. He was in a locked ward, which meant the same security as the state hospital, but the place itself wasn't as overbearing and there were more signs of life as day patients and visitors came and went. His medication continued, and Noel could resume his position as Paul's social worker and visit him regularly. As usual, I was at the end of the phone for Paul and the staff, if there were any concerns I could help with. Paul had a meeting with senior staff about three weeks after he'd settled in because they wanted to ask him about some of his beliefs and actions. They invited me to join them.

At the meeting, they questioned us about certain items that the police had taken from Paul's flat when they arrested him almost a year and a half before. One was a book, The Fred and Rose West story. They wondered why he would read such disturbing material. I had to admit that it had been my book. Previously Paul had chosen a few books from my bookcase and that was one of them. They seemed to think there might be something wrong with him reading troubling stories like that, but I didn't agree. I wouldn't have said this was unusual reading material, given that these types of books are in mass production and on shelves at every airport. To me, it was one of many appalling true crime stories that spark public interest.

Then they produced a few photographs from the police files. They focused on two to begin with. The first was of Paul standing with a rifle; he recognised it as one that had been taken in Germany. He wasn't on army duty as he was wearing casual clothes, and the background seemed to be a large meeting room or hall. They asked him to explain why he was holding a rifle and who had taken the photograph. He told them the army had allocated the weapon to him; however, he must have been breaking the rules by having it with him outside of his assigned duties. His best buddy had taken the photograph. They asked what his girlfriend, Dee, had had to say about him posing with a gun.

He replied, 'Let's see, shall we?' He turned the photograph over and we could see Dee had written some sort of love note on the back. They hadn't noticed that. He admitted he was wrong to be holding a gun and they accepted he wouldn't have been the only one making his own rules.

The next photograph was of a makeshift bomb in a box. This was a photograph I had taken a few Christmases beforehand. He was asked to tell them why he would want to build a fake bomb. He explained that the family members who were spending Christmas together had decided to give presents to be opened before Christmas dinner, but had been instructed to disguise them – the best one would win a prize. Paul had made an intricate structure out of marzipan and string with other odds and ends, all in a plain cardboard box; the final article looked like the real thing. He had cut out words from a newspaper, constructed a warning, stuck them on the lid of the box, then handed it to his Irish brother-in-law. Paul won the prize that day.

The photographs appeared to cause some concern amongst the medical team, but, in reality, there was nothing sinister about them. However, I could understand that if he had a propensity towards collecting items, photographs or books which implied murder and weapons, that needed to be addressed. They must have wondered where all this might end and how dangerous it could become when there were mental health issues involved. They didn't monitor Paul anymore because he had satisfied them with his answers; they never asked for another meeting like that.

However, two other concerns arose very soon after he arrived. First, Paul had brought his personal belongings from the state hospital; among them was a shaving kit. When the kit was found in his room, he was reprimanded because apparently shaving kits weren't allowed in patients' rooms. He said he wasn't aware of the details of the rules and thought they would be the same as the state hospital, but the staff said he should have asked. The psychiatrist told me he thought Paul was pushing the boundaries. The staff weren't happy with him at all; we did not need this.

Then, a few weeks later, I found out that they were extremely angry with Paul again and when I spoke to the psychiatrist on the phone, he told me in no uncertain terms that Paul was heading for trouble. My heart sank. A swastika sign had appeared on a piece of furniture in the common room attached to the ward. Paul, having had previous connections with Germany, was accused of carving out the sign which had badly damaged the leg of a chair. It hadn't been there before and it seemed more than coincidental that, as Paul had appeared, so had the swastika. The level of the doctor's anger was parallel with my level of disappointment. I remained calm, but I physically deflated.

I acknowledged his concern and all I could offer was, 'If Paul did this, then I don't know my son.'

I meant it. I could not imagine, given all that he'd been through, he would risk doing something as stupid as carving a sign on a chair. He had never shown a tendency towards Nazi views, so, if it had been him, his action was completely out of the blue. I asked where he would have got a knife or whatever he would have needed to make the sign, but, of course, no one knew. When I visited him, it came up in conversation.

Exasperated, he announced, 'Mum, what you've got to realise is that in a place like this, if you're accused of something, you just have to accept it.'

I asked him if he had done it.

He shook his head. 'No. And I've told them it wasn't me. What else can I do? They definitely think I'm to blame and that might mean I have to suffer.' He said that even if he knew who it was, it would be very difficult to convince the staff. I believed him.

I was pleasantly surprised when I called to arrange my next visit. One of the team members told me they had found out who had carved the swastika and it wasn't Paul. He apologised to me on behalf of the team. They had also spoken with Paul and admitted they had jumped to the wrong conclusion.

On my next visit he reminded me, 'You can't fight them. If they believe it, then they believe it. And there are more of them than me.'

He must have been reminded of his inability to deal with army superiors when he asked for help and had to accept that the word of those in authority is final. No negotiations allowed.

Despite those hiccups, little by little he continued to improve and, after a couple of months in the locked ward, he was transferred to an open ward. This meant he was allowed out to the hospital café. Then he was able to visit a nearby supermarket for a coffee. Very slowly, things were beginning to take shape.

However, yet another problem had to be addressed. Normally when a tenant vacates their council rental property for a year, the council have the right to take it back. Paul had been more than a year and a half between hospitals and the council started to ask questions despite the rent being paid up to date. I spoke with Noel and he agreed to support me if I wanted to appeal to the council. I told them although Paul had been away, he was now in the local hospital and would eventually come back to his flat. I also pointed out that if they evicted him, going through the application process again would mean they would have more work, they would have to give him a house anyway and the added stress would, without question, be detrimental to his health. Apart from the episode with the golf clubs, which they thankfully didn't know about, he had made a home. The property was clean and tidy and I was regularly checking things out and collecting mail. They agreed to allow him an extension as it seemed probable he would soon be able to return permanently to his flat.

When he was in the state hospital, the council had installed a new kitchen so things had improved since he first moved in. Before he went away, Paul had already repaired the damage to the walls and replaced most of the furniture so the place looked comfortable and liveable again, and the workers sent by the council did not notice any sign of his outburst. I made sure I was around at the same time as the workmen and I had taken photographs of his new kitchen so that he could see what he was coming back to. It had been a kind of incentive to keep his spirits up.

One afternoon, a few weeks after he had been transferred to the open ward, I collected him and asked if he'd like to see his flat, just a few streets away.

He looked at me wide-eyed then smiled. 'Yes, why not?'

I handed him his keys and we drove to the nearby car park. His hands were shaking but he was smiling as he opened his front door for the first time in a long time. He knew it was his flat, but after nearly two years, it must have seemed odd. Inside, he was disorientated. He was quiet and thoughtful as he looked at the kitchen then in each room and cupboard before stepping out onto the balcony. Then he went back into the kitchen for the tenth time and called out to me.

'Have you seen my new kitchen yet?' he joked.

We could have had a cup of tea but decided we would leave it until the next visit. We left, and I prayed that this would be another reminder that he had a life with us and could come back to it very soon. The social worker was a bit surprised that Paul had visited his flat but I didn't think we had acted too quickly. It was another goal for him to aim for.

Over time, he was trusted to leave the hospital for longer periods and even to spend a day with me at home. I would pick him up, take him to his own flat and leave him there. In the evening, I would collect him and make sure he got back to the hospital safely. He had to be back in the ward for his 9 pm curfew; if not, there would be repercussions.

One Sunday, I could pick him up, but I wasn't available to take him back, so he was responsible for the walk from his flat to the ward. When I saw him next, he told me the story of his trip back that night. He hadn't quite got his timing right and, halfway to the hospital, he realised that if he went all the way round to the entrance; he was going to be late. Not something he wanted in his notes. A high wall surrounded the hospital, and the only way he could get in was to climb over it. He did this, hoping that no police cars would pass by. It would have been difficult to explain why he was climbing INTO a psychiatric hospital. He also forgot that building works were going on inside the grounds and felt as if he was on an army training exercise as he scaled the wire fencing that blocked off the area being renovated, then ran like the wind to meet the deadline.

The next step in his recovery was when he could go back to his flat for a weekend initially, progressing to staying full time. Although his progress was encouraging, there was always the problem of him deciding to stop taking oral medication. They put the alternative suggestion of injections to him. It was worth a try, and he agreed.

I didn't have any doubt that Paul was ready to be released into the community, but that wasn't my decision to make. The positive outcome of the change in medication, coupled with optimistic regular reviews, convinced Dr Barrie that Paul could be discharged. He was pleased that he had accommodation in place and had resumed an interest in sports and getting himself an education.

Once he was at his flat permanently, Paul had a weekly outpatient appointment to have his injection and a short meeting with a medical team member. A good relationship had built up between Paul and the staff, especially with Bob, who administered his injections. Every so often, the staff asked him to give a urine sample. They tested it for drugs; the random tests were always clear. While he waited ten minutes for the results, there would be a bit of chat between them. After one of these tests, Bob came back to where Paul was waiting.

'I've got good news and bad news,' Bob whispered with a tilt of his head.

Paul looked at him with a quizzical expression.

Bob continued, 'The good news is you are drugs-free, but the bad news is… you're pregnant!' Humour was just as important to the staff as it was to us.

All was well, as Paul continued to put his life back together.

Chapter 21

Family Life

Things were taking shape. Once Paul was free of stays in hospital, Cait, John and I met with him each Sunday, alternating whose house we would use for Sunday dinner. These were lovely family times, and even if it was only Paul and me, we would still meet. After dinner, the two of us would watch a bit of TV or something that we had taped previously.

There was a time when Paul had recorded a documentary, although neither of us knew what the subject was. We settled down to watch it anyway. It started with the police responding to a call. A report had come in that a young man had barricaded himself in his flat and was angrily shouting from his window at no one in particular. Neighbours were concerned because he had brandished a machete and they thought he might have had other weapons inside. Armed police arrived and, for some time, tried to talk him down without success; he wouldn't even speak to them. They contacted his mother, who joined the police outside. She talked to her son as he stood at the window. The documentary showed her getting some dialogue going, reasoning with him and calming him down by reminding him of how they had solved other problems. He laid the machete down. Then the police interrupted the conversation and stopped her altogether, telling her she should leave because they could now deal with the situation. They took her away from the scene in a patrol car and, of course, her son saw her leave. The upshot was they couldn't get the same dialogue going with the young man, and he had picked up the machete again. When he was within their vision, the police shot him dead.

Paul looked at me. 'That'll be me someday, Mum.'

He had identified with the young man in the documentary, finding it difficult to trust and feeling no one understood what it was he was going through. It was a harrowing thought and somewhat disturbing.

Paul had celebrated his thirtieth birthday in the state hospital and, by the time he was thirty-one and back home, things were going well for him. Although he was still in contact with social services and regularly turning up for his injections, he was independent and led a fairly normal life. His income was stable. The council gave him an Access to Leisure card, which allowed him free entrance into leisure centres and pools. He went swimming with Cait and John and, if conditions were right, snowboarding with Andy, the friend he had met during his short stint at college. He had even bought a snowboard and the gear that went with it. He bought a computer and a mobile phone, as normal people do. A video camera and a costly Nikon camera followed soon after and he did a bit of photography.

Because his fascination with sticky tape and cardboard boxes as a boy had given way to toolboxes and wood, Paul decided he wanted to build a bar for his living room. He wasn't a drinker and I couldn't completely understand why he would want such an unusual piece of furniture. However, he had his mind set on it and over a few weeks, built himself quite an impressive corner bar, which was to become his domain. It was the perfect place to sit and watch TV while having a clear view over his balcony to the surrounding streets and car park. There were sections for this and sections for that in the bar, but he never had much alcohol in there as far as I could see. In a way, it could have been looked on as a divide between him and anyone else who came into the room.

His grandmother came to visit from further south and, perched on one of his barstools, she enjoyed a cup of tea with him. He took photos of her with his fancy camera and showed her how he could transfer them from the memory card to his computer, where her picture would miraculously appear on his television screen.

The months passed and we became a family again. We went to the cinema, out for meals, on trips to the countryside for barbeques and shopping for clothes or household items.

Well over a year had passed since Paul asked me to tell his father about the state hospital. It had ended there because Paul hadn't felt comfortable enough to take the next step. No communication had taken place between them since he left the house more than a decade before.

One afternoon, Paul's father had been in Aberdeen, en route to the airport. He was standing at a bus stop on a busy main road, speaking to his girlfriend on his mobile phone. As if in a movie, the throng of people around him parted slightly and amid them, he saw Paul, who had just come out of a supermarket. When his father finally found his voice, he suggested they go for a coffee. They made inroads into repairing what they could from a troubled relationship.

They exchanged numbers and promised to meet again. I thought Paul would be pleased that he had his 'hero' back in his life but, no, too much had happened.

'I don't know about all this. My dad wants to meet me and go swimming and do stuff like that. He's treating it as if we're old pals, but I can't forget what went on before. I don't mind seeing him sometimes, but I don't want him as a big part of my life.'

'Maybe you've got enough going on right now. You've got the family and Andy and a few pals. The main thing is you have people around that make you feel good. Only you know who these people are,' I volunteered.

What came back to me were comments from before; Cait saying he knew he had made a mistake when he went to stay with his dad at twelve years old and him telling me that as a teenager he felt his efforts at making things weren't appreciated. Whatever the truth was behind the blowup between him and his dad that had led to him being on the streets and his Red Book being withheld, I never really found out. I was convinced there were incidents that I would never know of that had caused an irreparable divide between father and son, but I was determined he would always have me to fall back on and live a settled life.

When *A Beautiful Mind* was showing at the local cinema, Paul and I went along to see it. There were a few scenes in the film where I held my breath, wondering what he would think about the protagonist experiencing delusional episodes. After the film, I asked what he thought of it all.

He replied, 'Well, that's what happens to you when you work for the secret service or the army. They're all out to get you and they win in the end.'

I thought it best to leave the conversation at that.

There was, however, always a reminder that Paul was under some form of care, either via an appointment with his social worker or a visit from the Community Psychiatric Nurse (CPN). The job of his CPN was to visit and check that his home life indicated he was able to survive without much additional input. It took some of the pressure away from me. I would have been looking for different things in him, but her trained eye would have picked up signs that perhaps I would not have noticed. When I spoke with her alone, she recounted the numerous cups of tea she took while sitting chatting to him; she spent longer in his flat than was probably necessary because she was intrigued by the stories of his life in Germany. He was happy to show her the things he had been doing to improve his flat. She told me she hardly ever sat down in some houses and had never accepted a cup of tea before. She didn't dare to drink from some of the cups or mugs she was offered for fear of catching some strange infection. Paul's ordered and extremely clean way of living didn't make her think twice. She was delighted with him and that made me feel good, so I told her a story that showed how proud I was to be a mother.

It happened one day after Paul had been released back to his flat full time and I was having coffee in town with Cait. As we sat looking out the café window, Paul walked by on the other side of the road. He wouldn't have heard us if we'd shouted because of the noise from the traffic. Cait called him on his mobile phone, and we watched him answering and turning around to come and join us. When we finished our coffees, we left. I was going one way as Paul and Cait were heading off in the opposite direction. We said our goodbyes and they walked off. After a minute I turned around – they had crossed the road and were walking away from me, together, brother and sister, and I was filled with so much pride and emotion I wanted to shout to the people who were walking past me and going about their busy lives,

Look, that's my son and my daughter! They're mine!

Probably this was a normal thing for parents to see but I couldn't remember having seen them walking together before, well, not as adults. I filled up with tears of happiness and watched them as they became lost in the crowd.

At one point, it struck me that in all the time Paul had been back with us, he had never expressed a wish to even visit his old haunts in central Scotland that had been his home for nearly six years before he joined the army. He'd gone there often enough while on army leave and had had plenty of opportunities since moving into his flat. He'd had enough money for bus or train fares and when he had his ambulance he could have driven there. But no, he never appeared to have any desire to catch up with anyone from that area.

I was pleasantly surprised when, around the end of summer 2005, Paul mentioned the possibility of going on holiday. Andy was now seriously involved with Debbie and a holiday with them wasn't quite what he was looking for. In any case, they were saving up for a wedding. Paul complained that he had no one to go on holiday with.

I put out the feelers. 'Well, for what it's worth, if you're happy to come with your old mother, we could go somewhere together.'

He didn't think sitting on a beach was for him, so we decided on a city break to Amsterdam over the New Year, and celebrate by bringing in 2006 in a different country. Paul had enjoyed Holland many times while on army leave as it wasn't too far from Germany, so we double-checked with his social worker who agreed that it would likely be a positive experience for us both. We booked a hotel on the outskirts of Amsterdam to make the best of a week there. Paul was certainly becoming more confident on his own in familiar territory, but he was still anxious about meeting new people. I was pretty sure he wouldn't be doing much on his own in Amsterdam.

With our two small flight bags, we set off on our journey. Checking into our hotel late in the evening meant we didn't see much except for the inside of the dining area. On our first day there, we set off to explore the area, where we soon found a nearby café and got chatting to the lady behind the counter. Her English was excellent and she introduced herself as Wilma; she was an extremely helpful lady who seemed to take Paul under her wing. She told us of pleasant restaurants, bus routes and places to visit.

On the second day, before we went into town, Paul suggested we drop into Wilma's again. He was soon chatting to her and some others who were having their morning coffee there. The seating was uncomfortable, in my opinion, where high bar stools contrasted with strange low chairs. I took my coffee to a window seat where I was more at ease. I sat watching Paul and his interactions with the others. It was good to see him taking part in everyday life.

The next morning he was ready first and told me he was going to Wilma's, suggesting I could meet him there when I was ready. I could have cried with joy. In only a few days, he had not only built up a trust with Wilma but also felt confident enough to walk out on his own.

We visited Madame Tussaud's, explored parks, went to flower markets and strolled down by the canals to see the boats. He became a regular at the café and Wilma even invited us to bring in the New Year there. We had lovely food and Paul relaxed in comfortable surroundings. It was a breakthrough. What Paul needed to restore his faith in life was: wings to fly, roots to come back to and reasons to stay. We had such a lovely time that when we came back to Scotland, we booked to go back in July; a summer holiday in Amsterdam was a trip to look forward to.

A couple of weeks later, Paul spoke about replacing his old TV. He had done a bit of research and said he'd seen a widescreen Sony TV in a shop but it cost nearly £2,000. He thought he couldn't justify spending that much on a TV so I suggested we go to the shop, have a look and ask what was on offer. We spoke about the fact that he had money saved and his entertainment was mainly through whatever he had at home. Was there any use in his money sitting in the bank? After much deliberation, he decided to buy the TV so we put it in the back of my car and drove home. He was looking forward to showing it off. However, when he got out of the car it struck him what he had done.

He announced, 'Mum, I'd ask you in for a cup of tea, but I need to go and lie down! I can't believe I've spent all that money. I need a rest!'

But I could see underneath he was a happy chappy. Good things were taking place. His grandmother visited again and he cleaned and scrubbed for her coming – he even cleaned out his freezer, as if she was going to inspect his frozen food! He was also looking forward to Andy's upcoming wedding. This was to take place in another city and he wanted to book a couple of nights in the same hotel where the reception was to be held.

The most exciting part of 2006 was one Sunday in March when we were having the usual lunch at my house. Cait and John announced to Paul and me that we would soon be welcoming a new baby into the family. Looking at the scan we were overjoyed. The due date was September. This was something neither Paul nor I had ever thought about or discussed so, between us all, we had a few funny one-liners about grandmothers and uncles. It was wonderful news and Paul and I spoke about the baby each time we met.

However, something must have been niggling at Paul because, not long after the wonderful announcement, he said, 'Mum, I've got something to tell you. I've got a funny feeling I'll never get to look after this baby.'

His comment made the hairs on the back of my neck stand up, but I tried to reassure him. 'Well, I'll be here with you so we can look after the baby together.'

I knew where he was coming from. Even though he was doing very well, there were always clouds hanging over him that would make other people extremely uncomfortable: the gun, the violence and his stay in psychiatric hospitals. His being around children would have been out of the question for most parents. At the back of my mind was the time Susie had let him hold baby Cameron.

Her words came flooding back to me, 'Who knows, he might never get another chance in life to hold a baby.' I hoped with all my heart this wouldn't be the case and that he wouldn't blot his copybook again.

Easter was drawing close, and he kept an eye on school holidays because he knew that's when I wouldn't be working. He called me a few days before the Easter break began and queried, 'Mum, am I right, are you on holiday for the next two weeks?'

I told him I certainly was, and he jumped in with, 'Wicked! That means we'll be able to go somewhere different for coffee.'

I went to visit him on the morning of Easter Sunday and we put the world to rights. He'd no plans for the rest of the day and as I was leaving, we chatted at his front door.

Jokingly, I scolded him, 'Look at you. It's a lovely day, the kind of day for going out!'

He stepped over the threshold onto the street, then quickly jumped back inside and in a cheeky voice announced, 'Look, I've *been* out!'

There was nothing at all unusual about that day and I can't explain why, but when I left him, I let out an enormous sigh. And so the Easter holiday began.

Chapter 22

The Shock

The following day was a splendid Easter Monday; I went to visit friends who were holidaying outside the city. Newly arrived from Canada, they looked forward to taking in the beauty of the Scottish Highlands. As we drove through picturesque towns and villages into the countryside, we chatted about family. When we stopped at a café, their three children jumped out, laughing at the cows in the fields and squealing with delight as they hurried towards the stream that ran close by. Throwing pebbles into the water, they reminded me so much of family life when Paul and Cait were younger. As we relaxed and watched the children play, I formed a plan for later in the week. This beautiful setting with spectacular views, the smell of fresh fields and the sound of the odd animal would be the perfect place to bring Paul. He could drive and we would take in the sights, sample the scrumptious home baking and enjoy some quality time together.

On Tuesday, I called Paul to tell him of my plan, but there was no reply either from his mobile or his landline, so I left a message and suggested we pay a visit to the new area I had discovered. Around 8 pm I called for a second time, but once again there was no reply. Remembering that his favourite programme would be on, I left it. He had already announced that he didn't answer the phone during *The Bill* or *Fifteen to One*.

I called again early on Wednesday. I felt as though I could be bothering him, but it simply wasn't like him not to reply to my message. I tried calling again later, but there was no answer. This time, his mobile phone went directly to voicemail. I decided that I'd have to arrive unannounced at his door the next day if only to double-check.

The next morning, Thursday, I called another twice, but there was still no answer. I picked up his spare key and thought, *I hope I don't have to use this.*

I could have put money on the knowledge that he would not have grabbed a bag and disappeared again. The upcoming arrival of the new baby had animated him. He had often repeated the same lines, 'Mum, you don't know how excited I am. I'm going to be an uncle!'

I went through different scenarios, most highly unlikely, but maybe he had just made a last-minute visit to some old haunts. Maybe he and a friend had taken off somewhere and his mobile might not be picking up a signal.

To a certain extent, this had happened a few months before with Andy. At the start of the year, they had headed into the mountains for an overnight stay, a bit of trekking and some sightseeing. I had been visiting Susie when they set off one bitter day and, as she lived in the country, I stayed over to avoid a drive home in the dark. It had been exceptionally cold, and I woke a few times during that January night thinking about Paul and Andy. In the morning I said to Susie, 'I was thinking about them, out there in the freezing cold. I hope they're OK.'

She had tried to encourage me by pointing out how young and fit they were. 'Oh, they'll be fine. They'll be snuggled up in a bothy somewhere with their camping stove to keep them warm.' I hadn't been convinced that they'd even taken a stove, never mind being in a bothy.

A couple of days after that trip with Andy, Paul recounted the story of their adventure that winter night. They had tried to cross a river, fallen in and got soaked in the ice-cold water. They had no way of drying themselves, and Paul suddenly acted strangely. He was talking rubbish and falling about. Andy, fortunately, was more on the ball; he had his mobile phone and called his father, who drove for over an hour to get to them. When he arrived, he realised the guys were suffering from hypothermia. After calling an ambulance, he tried his best to do what he could for them. Once the emergency services arrived, they wrapped Paul and Andy in what was described to me as strong silver paper, loaded them into the ambulance and took them to hospital. They discharged Andy, but kept Paul in overnight. It amazed me that such an escapade could have taken place while I was completely ignorant of what was going on. It could be the same this time. Just lads wanting an adventure.

So, as I tried to contact Paul that Thursday, I consoled myself that it wasn't beyond the realms of possibility they had taken off again. However, this time, although I envisaged him getting involved in something where he'd lost track of time, my heart and mind were extremely unsettled.

Andy was a city traffic warden and, on my way to Paul's flat, I saw a traffic warden across the street. Parking my car in a no-parking zone, I called him over, knowing I'd get his attention. He'd likely be ready to give me a scolding. As he approached, I could only begin with, 'Listen, I know this is going to sound crazy, but I haven't been able to get in touch with my son for the last few days and I think you might help. My son's friend is Andy. He's a traffic warden. Do you know Andy?'

He stepped back, smiling. 'Andy? Of course, I know Andy; I trained him for this job.'

I asked him if there was any way he could find out if Andy had taken holidays, because that might explain why Paul was not answering his phone.

He took out his handheld machine and said, 'Of course I can tell you. I can look right here to see who's on duty and who's not.' After a quick scroll through, he announced, 'OK, I can see his timetable here. But Andy is on duty right now. He's in the city centre with another colleague.'

Feelings of disappointment and confusion washed over me as I let out a sigh of exasperation, but I thanked him anyway.

He tried to reassure me, 'I'm sure your son is fine. I hope you find him soon. Take care.'

As I got back in the car I realised our conversation had raised more questions than answers. Parking in the car park near Paul's flat, I looked up at his windows. Everything looked more or less normal although the bedroom curtains were closed. Maybe he was having a long lie. I rang the bell and rapped on his door several times but there was no answer. The silence after each ring and knock was deafening. Eventually, I knocked on a couple of neighbours' doors to ask if they had seen Paul.

One woman who lived directly below him said, 'No, we haven't. Usually, Paul takes the bins in and he hasn't done it this week. We haven't heard or seen him for a few days. Is everything OK?'

I said I was sure it was but I was concerned because he hadn't been in touch with me or answered my calls. With my heart in my mouth, I took his key out of my bag and, despite my shaking hand, somehow placed it in line with the lock. It refused to go in; there was a key on the other side. There are no words to describe how I felt, probably numb. I had a feeling this wasn't going to have a good outcome. Someone was inside, someone had locked the door and that someone wasn't answering. I needed help and the only people I could think of were the police.

As my stomach churned, I managed to drive to the nearby local station and spoke to a policewoman at the desk. I told her the story and said that four days had passed since I'd spoken to Paul – maybe not unusual for any other young man but quite unusual for him. The policewoman asked for some personal details: his age, his address and suchlike. I really needed her attention and mentioned that, in the past, there had been a gun involved. She asked if I thought that might be the case now.

I replied without hesitation, 'Absolutely not.'

I explained that the immediate neighbours hadn't seen him and that I couldn't open his door. She left me for a few minutes then came to tell me that a unit would be at Paul's flat in half an hour and asked if I wanted to be there.

'Yes, I'll be there, waiting in my car.' I added, 'I hope I'm sending you on a wild goose chase and that you find him surrounded by twelve lassies!' I guess, more than anything, such a remark was a way of keeping my own spirits up.

By the time I got back to Paul's flat, there was a strange toy wedged in the letterbox. It was a hard, plastic

SpongeBob SquarePants. I had no idea what that was about but I took it out and put it in my bag. I rang the bell again in the hope that something had transpired since I'd left and that SpongeBob might hold the key. Still no answer.

I spent the longest half hour of my life waiting for official help. There were no new thoughts, only an emotionless detachment from the ordinary things that were happening in the street. A few people coming and going, the odd car leaving and the postman making his rounds.

The police unit arrived exactly when they said they would, a WPC and a PC. I couldn't wait a moment longer. Before they were out of the patrol car, I approached them. The PC asked me to confirm that I was the mother of the person whose flat we were heading to; he clarified Paul's name. He asked if Paul might use a nickname with friends, which he didn't and, as we stood outside the door, he enquired about the layout of the flat. I told them that behind Paul's front door there was a flight of stairs. These led to a normally unlocked door that opened into the main hall and living areas. He seemed satisfied with what I'd told him.

The PC rang the bell, then shouted Paul's name several times through the letterbox.

He called out, 'Paul, Paul, this is the police. If you're inside, you'll need to give us some signal or we are going to come in.'

There was no movement from inside, only the same deafening silence as before.

Again the PC spoke through the letterbox, 'Paul, Paul, this is the police. If you don't let us know that you're inside we'll have to break your door down. Now!'

Again, no movement or sound from inside. I told the PC that all that was holding the door shut, apart from the key in the lock, was a small, sliding snib about three-quarters of the way up. With a couple of powerful kicks, the door flew open. He told me to wait exactly where I was while they both climbed the stairs.

They continued calling out, 'Paul, Paul, Paul! Paul, are you there? It's the police here.'

Moments later, I heard the PC give a short cough and I knew he had found something. I started up the stairs but only got halfway when the PC met me. He put his hand out to stop me and said, 'OK, there's someone in the bedroom. We found a male, and he's dead. He's lying in the bed and appears to have been there for some time.'

For four days, I had had negative nigglings. It was only on that morning that I hadn't been able to drag any positive reasons from the universe as to why Paul wasn't responding. My intuition told me something serious had happened, but the worst I could come up with was that he had done something stupid, although I couldn't think what, and couldn't fix it. If the notion of his death even flitted into my mind, somehow my brain wouldn't let it linger. When I heard the policeman's words, I can only describe my mind's reaction as brain freeze. There seemed to be a movement inside my head like electric sparks or fireworks, but there were no thoughts, only the words *male* and *dead* remained of the PC's sentence.

All that came out of my mouth was, 'I need to see.'

I would have said I became a statue, riveted to the spot, but I couldn't have been because I found myself at the top of the stairs. As I headed for the bedroom, the PC walked in front, turning around a few times, keeping his eye on me. My heart was racing and my mouth was dry as I looked into the bedroom. There, lying face down on the bed, was Paul.

Lifeless. He was covered with his quilt. Well, everything except for his enormous feet dangling over the end of the bed.

All I could manage in a quiet voice was, 'Oh, Paul.'

The WPC ushered me into the living room where I sat down. After a few seconds, I seemed to absorb the initial shock and my mind let reality filter in. I shook uncontrollably and was oblivious to most of what was going on around me.

As I came back down to earth, I could answer what seemed to me to be endless questions. I heard the PC contacting the station and the WPC asking if there was someone they could get in touch with to come over to be with me. The only person I could think of was my son-in-law, John. The WPC called him at work, only telling him there had been an incident at Paul's flat and asking if he could come over immediately.

Time seemed to stand still one minute, then race the next; nature had a wonderful way of taking me out of the moment. *Frozen in time* doesn't fully describe how my mind and body reacted to such severe shock. Somehow, the inability to think straight combined with automatic reactions allowed the shock to dissipate a bit at a time. Slowly, the reality of the here and now sank in, then alternated with disbelief before finally, for me at least, giving way to… what happens next?

I looked around and saw signs of the routine Paul adhered to. His television magazine was open at the previous Monday's TV listings, something that he ritually did at night before going to bed. This meant he had turned the page to Monday at some point the previous Sunday after I had left him. The only thing in the bin was one small, empty beer bottle. His kitchen was tidy, with no cups or plates to be seen. Paul had arranged the bathroom towels properly and nothing at all was out of place. No evidence of anyone else having been in the flat. The police continued with their notebooks in hand, asking a mountain of questions.

The flat was filling with various people. To add to the melee, there was a forensic detective and a doctor inside and an officer who stood guard on the street outside the main door. I only knew this because I heard Andy's voice somewhere in the background, so I put my head around the corner, looked down the stairs and told the officer it was OK for Andy to come up. He was stunned when he heard what we had found. My son-in-law arrived and introduced himself to the officer at the door; he climbed the stairs to learn that Paul was dead.

At one point, I mentioned the SpongeBob SquarePants toy and Andy said he was the one who had tried to put it through the letterbox. He had been trying to contact Paul for days on his mobile and realised when his calls went straight to voicemail that something was wrong. The toy was a bit of a joke between them and he thought if Paul had a problem and wasn't answering to anyone, the toy would be a sign, he'd know that Andy was around to help. Then Andy revealed he had been a hair's breadth away from kicking in the door himself. One policeman straightened up and reminded Andy that if he'd done that, Paul's flat would have become a crime scene and Andy would have had lots of questions to answer. I wouldn't have been able to go in and identify Paul, and Andy's actions could have denied me entry to the flat for a long time. Thankfully, the police had beat Andy to it.

The WPC took me out of the room and whispered that they were about to turn Paul over on the bed, and after that, he would be taken away. I asked if I could see him once more and when he was face up I went into the bedroom, where yet another PC was. I didn't realise at the time, but that was me officially identifying Paul. He was indeed my son and not some stranger. I looked around his bedroom and saw his clothes, jeans and a jumper, neatly folded on a chair. Again there are no words to describe the feelings I had. Shock, sadness and confusion don't even come close. I left him there and went back to the living room in the knowledge that my role as a mother to Paul was now over.

The sounds that filtered through from the bedroom were probably a stretcher or a gurney being brought in and out. I chose not to look but only to imagine. I had to leave him in the capable hands of the people who were going to carry him down the stairs and out of his flat for the last time.

Noel, Paul's social worker, had to be told. I didn't know what the grapevine was like, but I wanted to speak to him personally and tell him before he found out by chance. My call was put through immediately and as usual, his cheery greeting was welcomed.

Unsure of my voice, I questioned him, 'Noel, I take it you are sitting down?'

'Oh yes, as always! And how are things with you today?' he enquired.

I couldn't answer as my throat seemed to narrow and I felt a rise of panic. I thought I was choking as I tried to swallow. I finally managed to react, my voice shaking. 'I'm in Paul's flat and I've got some very sad news.' I had started to get some words out so, without pausing for breath, I rambled on. 'We've found Paul in his bed and he's dead. By my calculations, he's been there since Sunday night, but that still has to be confirmed. I've been told there don't appear to be any suspicious circumstances, but that's all I know except that there doesn't seem to have been anyone else in the flat with him.'

Then I breathed again.

Noel was in shock and arranged to call me back once he had processed what I'd told him. As a city social worker, he would have heard sad and devastating stories and been involved in many instances of losing clients. Much later, he told me that for the first time in his life, he'd been so affected by the news of Paul that he had to leave the building because he was crying. He got someone else to deal with his next few appointments.

Chapter 23

And Finally

In the midst of all this chaos and people coming and going, my mobile phone rang. When I looked at the caller display I could see the call was from Paul's grandmother, now in her eighties. Everyone was quiet as I took the call. She was coming up to the area soon and had arranged to visit Paul, but something had changed and she wasn't going to make it on the day they had planned so she wanted to change the day. She'd been trying to get in touch with Paul for a couple of days but couldn't. She asked if I'd tell him she'd see him later.

All I could manage was, 'OK, I'll tell him.'

I pulled myself together and asked her how she was, but I knew my voice was far from normal. She told me she was looking forward to coming up to see us, then we hung up. Our conversation was more abrupt than normal. I had no more to say. With no one by her side, I couldn't have told her that she had called a few moments after her grandson had left home for the final time.

We were also concerned about Cait, who was nearly four months pregnant by this time. She was on a shopping trip and my son-in-law asked if I'd come back to their house with him to be there when she returned, but first, he had to return to work to ask for some time off.

Gradually, Paul's flat started to empty of people. The numbness I felt when I locked his door that day was probably nature's way of allowing me to carry on in automatic pilot.

Cait returned and was told the shocking news about her brother. We joined forces, cried on and off, and sat around in disbelief. At one point I realised Paul was right, he would never get to look after the baby.

The next day I contacted an aunt and uncle who were, by sheer coincidence, making their way over to see Paul's grandmother. I told them I'd call once they'd arrived and also what I'd be telling her. When I broke the news to her, she dropped the phone. I couldn't be with her, but at least she had someone there to console her.

A few hours later, I knew I would have the job of telling Paul's father. I dialled his number, only to discover from his girlfriend that he was offshore and wasn't due back for another two weeks. She kindly got in touch with his boss and he flew Paul's father home immediately.

They took Paul to the mortuary and the procurator fiscal's office became involved because this was the sudden death of what appeared to be a healthy, thirty-one-year-old man. They were to perform an autopsy to decide what had happened, but there was no telling when the results of that would be available.

It looked as if Paul had been alone when he took his last breath. There was nothing to show it had been a homicide. Also, the progress he had made with the care system and how much he was looking forward to being an uncle told me there was absolutely no way he had taken his own life.

He was no longer the hopeless, starving young man with no support in Germany. I spoke with the procurator fiscal's office several times as they tried to determine what the cause of death was. They carried various tests, but each day brought the same answer.

'No news yet.'

Young people rarely die in bed asleep, and the mystery surrounding his passing was tough to contend with. After informing friends and family that Paul was no longer with us, we had to think about a funeral, but it was difficult to give a day and time without Paul's body being released.

Waiting for news gave us time to reflect more on the events of the previous few years. During the four years since I had brought Paul back from Germany, he'd had about eighteen months in his house before spending roughly another eighteen months between the state hospital and the local hospital. My calculations told me he had had a year on the outside with us before he had passed away. It all seemed so cruel and unfair and there was no rescuing him now.

I had contacted some of his friends in Germany and told them we were expecting to hold the funeral the following week. They made plans to visit. Four shocked friends, two young men and two young women, came over to Scotland for four days. During their stay, we spoke at length about Paul's life in and out of the army and between the photographs they had brought and what I had, we were able to piece together a part of his life that I hadn't known about.

One of the young women seemed to know lots about Paul and, amongst other stories, she told me about one night when Paul had come back to the flat he shared with some friends. He had slept on the sofa and in the morning when she saw him, he was foaming at the mouth. It wasn't much, it was only trickling down his chin, but enough to alarm her. She mentioned it to him when he woke up, but he seemed to dismiss it. Although this incident had occurred years before the gunshot wound or his recent course of medication, I thought I should inform the procurator fiscal.

When I told him he said, 'Actually, this ties in with what we think we've found.'

They had detected some sort of seizure. This was news to me; I had never witnessed evidence of him having had a fit as a child and, apart from what his friend revealed about a trickle of foam, what had caused his passing was impossible for the procurator fiscal to tell. I couldn't help but think that his injury, meningitis and surgery may have added to an existing condition.

I took the four friends to Paul's flat and we sat for a while. I told them he had made the bar and they took turns sitting on his barstool, making comments about how he would have felt like the king of the castle sitting so high up. One of the things I mentioned was that Paul wasn't always comfortable going out without his hat, and I wondered what they made of that. The guys nodded. That was the Paul they knew, always wearing a hat when he could. Speaking about it reminded me of a time when I'd mentioned it to Paul.

I recounted his story. 'You know something? In the army, the soldiers wear hats but never when they're eating or in the mess with the others. It's an unspoken rule. If a soldier doesn't want anyone to speak to him for any reason, he keeps his hat on. That's a sign that he wants to be left alone and everyone respects that. Even if he's sitting having his food. No one asks him to take his hat off and he's left at peace to deal with whatever is going on.'

The two young men looked at me, smiled and nodded. It was true; a respectful gesture between soldiers. I was glad I had never discouraged Paul from wearing his hat, no matter if others thought it was rude. There had been a story behind his actions.

His friends weren't surprised at his tidiness and told me stories of when he'd shared flats, how he had become frustrated at the messiness of other people. I pointed out some pictures on the walls that Paul had painted and, despite being surprised at how well done they were, they laughed as they joked about times he'd used paint before. They'd tried to decorate a mate's house and it seems more paint ended up on the floor than the walls. They'd given up and gone for a beer, they reckoned the poor mate's house would still be in the same state.

After a while, I said I was going to leave them together in Paul's flat. I told them I wanted to take a walk to give them time to take in what feelings and emotions they could from Paul's special place without me intruding. Theirs had been an exceptional time together, their friend was gone and this was the only opportunity they would have to say goodbye. The young woman who had talked about his mouth foaming gave me a letter she had written for Paul and asked me to put it in his casket. It transpired she was the one who had written the letter in German to him when he was in the state hospital, but at that time she didn't know he wasn't at home. Maybe they'd had a relationship at some time, I will never know.

Sadly, no funeral took place while they were there. The four took themselves back off to Germany but left me with some lovely stories and memories. Soon after they'd gone, I got word that Paul's body would be released within a few days, so we could start to think about a date for a service and closing down his flat for good.

After Cait and I divided up things like his cameras, television and some pictures, I contacted the few friends Paul had and told them that they were more than welcome to take something of Paul's if they wanted. The odd ashtray or bottle opener was enough for them. His grandmother took his mobile phone as a reminder of her only grandson who was taken too soon. I kept his cutlery and still use it to this day. It reminds me that he finally got the opportunity to build up a house, complete with a kitchen and cupboards full of food, where he could fulfil the basic needs of sustenance, warmth and rest.

While I was at his flat tidying out some belongings, one friend, Peter, appeared at the door saying he'd like to take something. He came in and we sat chatting for a while. I was sure he wanted to say something but didn't quite know how to; he seemed to be holding back.

They'd met not long after Paul arrived in the city, about four years before. Peter had been born and bred there. I knew the area he lived in; famous for its shady characters, and no doubt he told Paul stories about some of the hair-raising incidents that had taken place. As we spoke, my suspicions about his discomfort became certain as he broached the subject of guns.

He bravely mentioned, 'I know Paul was in the army and used rifles and suchlike, but I've got something to tell you and something to ask you.'

He proceeded to tell me that, a while before, during a discussion about weapons, Paul had asked him if he could get his hands on a gun. Peter had been taken aback by this request.

While I was listening intently, he continued, 'I think Paul was going a bit nuts.'

I replied, 'In a way, it doesn't surprise me that he was making enquiries about a gun and if he'd got his hands on one, who knows what might have happened?'

Then Peter leaned forward. 'So, now my question. Later, Paul told me he'd shot himself. That's not true, is it?'

I had to tell him, 'Yes, Peter. It's true. Unbelievable, but entirely true.'

He sat back with a shudder. If he had been surprised by Paul's request for a gun, he was even more shocked to hear that shooting himself had indeed been a part of Paul's past. He hadn't believed Paul and may well have scoffed or shown some signs of horror when Paul had told him. One thing was sure; he'd thought Paul was going crazy at one point.

I had another task before me. We had planned to go back to Amsterdam in the summer. With our flights booked and, because Paul had enjoyed the location of the hotel and Wilma's café, we had put a deposit on the same accommodation as before. Our travel and the hotel had to be cancelled; I wouldn't have gone on my own. It would have been too sad. I wrote to Wilma and told her Paul was no longer with us, and it delighted me that she took the time to write back and send her condolences.

Eventually, I had a call from the procurator fiscal to say Paul was being released to the undertakers the next day. They completed and signed the necessary certificate and the cause of death read, 'Probable Epileptic Seizure'. With that part of the process over, the following day I met with the undertaker to arrange a date for a service. He said I should think about the clothes I might want Paul to wear and that I should bring them immediately. I went straight to his flat and looked out his beige chunky jumper, along with a pair of jeans and, of course, his matching beige woolly hat. When I dropped them off, I asked when I could see Paul again.

The undertaker said, 'If you or anyone else wants to see him, you'll have no choice but to come back later today. He's showing signs of deterioration and we need to seal the casket by the end of the day.'

Because of distance and timing, no one else, not even his father, could go, but I went back around 6 pm. I could see there were changes; he had very few eyelashes left. I stood for a while looking at him, shaking my head in disbelief. How could this be? I took in as much as I could – his face, his hair, his jumper – then I noticed his hat. The undertaker had dressed Paul but, rather than put his hat on his head, he had folded it and placed it between his hands; he was holding his woolly hat. Somehow it seemed a mark of respect. I have often thought of that kind gesture.

As I slipped two notes from his cousins and the letter from his German friend down the side of the casket, I looked at my son for the last time. I kissed his cold forehead and all I could say was, 'Bye Paul.'

Epilogue

The next time I drove to Paul's flat I felt dreadful knowing he wouldn't be there. No longer was I to be filled with the expectation of drinking tea, chatting and laughing with him. I was deflated and empty. Driving past what had previously been insignificant buildings and shops that had been taken for granted, I started to see them in a different light.

Thoughts like, *He won't ever feel as if he's walking on air down that street, he can't drive on this road again, he won't shop there anymore and he'll never appear around that corner.*

Walking towards his door, knowing that inside were only *things* reminded me of how unimportant material goods were, but these were Paul's things and that made them precious.

As I opened the door, I found myself paying attention to the light-coloured carpet that climbed the stairs before me. I thought about how bright the hall was when all the doors were open. I deliberately took in the smell of his flat; I'd never noticed the intricate design on his favourite plant pot that was sitting, lonely, on the table. With a new set of eyes, I took in all the things he loved but would never be able to look at or touch again. The barstool, the kettle, the TV listings.

After I surveyed the other rooms, it was with a kind of reverence I took a step into his bedroom. Standing at the foot of the bed, tears rolled down to my chin. Somehow, I could feel his contentment as he got ready for bed that Easter Sunday night. He'd have been happy that he'd pottered around all day, drank numerous cups of tea and watched a bit of TV while sipping on his cold beer and smoking a cigarette. Finally, after having a sneak preview at what was on TV the following day and placing his remote controls in their exact spot on his bar, he'd have switched everything off and double-checked all the electrical sockets. Brushing his teeth would have been the last thing he'd have done before finally going into his bedroom. He might have checked the computer on his desk immediately inside the door, or maybe not. After meticulously folding his clothes and making sure everything was exactly as he wanted it, he would have, unwittingly, lain down and closed his eyes for the last time in the bed I was now standing before.

Seeing the pillow where he last rested his head made me feel strangely warm inside. I remembered the pillow that had comforted baby Paul as he rested in his cot, the Action Man pillow which had given him such pleasure as a boy, the oversized pillow which had supported Paul the man as he lay confused in Göttingen University Hospital, and in that moment I experienced an overwhelming urge to let my face touch the pillow he'd gone to sleep on, forever. So, I lay down, only for a moment.

Paul's flat had to be emptied and returned to the council. Some family members came to help and took what they felt they could. The bar that Paul had made had been especially significant – that was his corner of the living room where he could survey everything that had been important to him. I'd watched the delight it had given him as it took shape, the bits of wood forming shelves and dividers, the top sanded down several times and varnished and the beading carefully placed around the outer edges. He had built it in the living room, but it hadn't been assembled in sections and couldn't be taken out. The narrow door and turn of the stairs meant there was no alternative but to pull it apart and dispose of it. That wasn't an operation I could easily watch, so I left the flat while some others did the necessary. Of course, on my return, there was a huge, visible gap in the living room, but not as much of a gap as I would feel for the rest of my life.

A framed picture of a pretty Scottish scene sat above Paul's sofa, but no one had a use for it. Thinking it might be a friendly gesture to take it up to the hospital where Paul had had his weekly injections, I made an appointment to see Bob. I put the picture in the boot of the car and headed off. Bob spoke fondly of Paul then revealed a few things that made me realise he was carrying some guilt. As I pushed him further, he wept, saying he wondered if he'd made a mistake with Paul's last injection and that he had contributed to Paul's death. I reassured him that couldn't possibly be the case; the autopsy had revealed nothing untoward. The procurator fiscal had been aware of all the treatment Paul was receiving and everything had checked out. Nothing legal or illegal had been in his system that could have caused his death.

I told Bob Paul had thought a lot of him. 'He called you a good guy… for what that's worth!'

We laughed. Bob was visibly relieved. The poor man had even spoken to his superiors about his fears, wondering if the family would blame him. Finally, I told him what I had in the boot and he was honoured to take it, saying he'd make sure Paul's picture would have pride of place in the ward.

There were some surplus pieces of furniture by the end of the clear-out. I contacted a community charity who agreed to uplift what remained. They seemed surprised at the items going to charity. When they heard the story, they were amazed that a young man in his early thirties, living alone into the bargain, had kept the place so clean and tidy. I told them that hadn't always been the case and joked about his life as a messy kid but said that the army had made a huge difference.

One of them responded, 'Can I just say, when we are invited to empty a young person's home it's sometimes because they've died as a result of substance abuse. You have no idea what we find and what we've got to deal with. I can tell you now, looking at this place, your son was a clean-living young man.'

My maternal pride was obvious by the grin on my face. I also felt I'd grown in height.

Another insight into Paul's mind was uncovered when I gave his desk and swivel chair to a colleague. It was a reasonably sized corner desk. Her son dismantled it into manageable parts and loaded it into his van. Once I was back at work a few weeks later, she asked if I'd come into her office. When they'd been reassembling the desk, they'd found some documents taped to the underside of a drawer. There was a duplicate passport with Paul's name and picture, plus a copy of his birth certificate. Paul always had the means to grab the essentials at the last minute and get away without being traced. That saddened me. He could have vanished in a heartbeat.

On the day of the funeral service, the hearse drew up outside my house and we made our way into the car behind. The gesture of one undertaker was pleasantly surprising. He stopped the traffic and walked in front of the hearse until the cortège arrived at traffic lights a few feet away. It was as if we forced the rest of the world to slow down and pay their respects to Paul. At the funeral home, it was such a delight to see so many friends, family and colleagues from near and far. The majority had never even met Paul, but their support was invaluable. Noel, Dr Barrie, Bob and some of the medical team kindly rearranged their busy schedule to attend the service at the crematorium. The entrances to both chapels of rest there were open. As we drew up to the crematorium, we were directed to the first entrance, but I noticed a vaguely familiar figure hovering outside the second entrance.

There were no flowers except that close family each had a lily and, one by one, we laid them on Paul's coffin as we passed by to take our seats. I noticed his father and girlfriend sitting in the front row on the other side of us. It was a sad sight as it was now too late for real amends to be made between him and his only son. My cousin led the brief service and, as was normal, Paul's casket sat in front of the gathering.

After my cousin had spoken about life and death, crying and grieving, he said, 'And now Paul's mum is going to say something.'

A few people around me gasped. It may have been unusual for someone so close to the person who had passed away to speak, but I was together enough and determined to say my piece about my boy. I stood up and walked over to the side of Paul's casket which was raised on a plinth. I knew I had done the right thing when I started by addressing the congregation and didn't dissolve. 'Paul means the Little One and so today I'd like to say something to my little one.'

Then I turned to look at his casket.

'Paul, I want to say thanks for being in my life. I especially want to say thanks for some things that have brought a smile to my face. When you were about five years old, you loved to get your hands on a screwdriver and ended up taking things apart to see what was inside.' With a bit of a smile, I added, 'Thanks for assuring me you could rebuild them.' I continued, 'When you were a little bit older and Santa brought you your BMX bike, you said I was the best mum in the world. Thanks for saying that, because then I knew you didn't believe in Santa Claus. Another time I wanted to buy a car. You were eager to help me decide which one was right for me. Thanks for your help, although I quickly realised you'd chosen the kind of car that *you* wanted to drive.'

Then I climbed the two steps of the plinth so that I could rest my hand on his casket and, keeping it there, I continued. 'And Paul, when times were tough for you and you thought you weren't going to make it, we joined forces and you pulled through. Thanks for trusting me.' Then I stepped down and finished with, 'And thanks for being MY little one.'

As I walked away from Paul, I knew these would be the last words I would direct at him and I was grateful that I had been strong enough to speak to him one more time. I sat down with the others in time to watch his casket slowly disappearing forever through two small red velvet curtains.

I learned later that there were two funerals on at the same time in the different chapels and the man who had been hovering outside the second door had been Dr Simons. He'd ended up going to the wrong funeral. Ironically, he was the doctor who, at a meeting, scolded Paul and me for laughing about Tony Blair talking to Paul through the TV. I hope he saw the funny side of paying his last respects to someone he didn't know.

A few days before the service, I had gone to Paul's flat, intending to clear out some paperwork. I found information relating to the Save the Children organisation. I found what looked like a copy of a direct debit form, which told me that he was donating money every month to the charity. I was very impressed and thought it a commendable thing. I remembered he'd spoken about it but I didn't realise he was participating. As there were to be no flowers at his service, I had contacted Save the Children and asked if we could have some envelopes to leave for people who might want to donate, given that this was a charity close to Paul's heart. In the end, the small congregation had donated well over £400. A lovely gesture.

A few days later I contacted the charity again to tell them and arranged to pass over the collection. A kind man listened to my story and, as I spoke, he looked up Paul's name on his computer records. I indicated that I was surprised that Paul hadn't told me he was donating to their charity.

He volunteered, 'Well, to be honest, I'm not surprised he didn't tell you, because this is the strangest thing ever. We had an enquiry from him not that long ago and all the paperwork was completed but for some strange reason we've never taken the donation from his account, not a penny!'

I couldn't help but laugh to myself. *What else could possibly have gone wrong in Paul's life?*

However, I told the man that this would be a little surprise for Save the Children and arranged to send a cheque. I received a heartwarming letter in reply. Paul wasn't able to save the children in Bosnia, but I can only hope that the small contribution from those who attended his funeral somehow made a child's life a bit better, if even for a day.

Paul had gone from having absolutely nothing in Germany to having a comfortable home in Scotland, a few decent pieces of technology, some nice clothes and money in the bank. He had been living a good life, not extravagant, but not like the distressed pauper he once was. Thanks to the support he had from the hospital staff, his mental health issues were under control. The army had also helped by relieving any financial worries, but his progress was not only to do with what he received through pensions but also by watching how other people lived. He had admired Cait and John and took many cues from them about living within one's means. He also learned that success was not of value if measured by external material possessions.

As a family, although we hadn't many material things, we had made last wills and testaments and Paul had decided he'd like to do the same. We gave him a rough idea of the kind of things he might want to think about before visiting the solicitor, for example, he would be expected to ask someone he trusted to be his executor and then think about how he'd like any possessions or money to be distributed. He had given it some consideration and asked his brother-in-law, John, if he would be his executor. He said that Cait and I would be the beneficiaries of all his worldly possessions. The only other thing he considered important and wrote into his will was that, if anything happened to him, he'd like there to be a memorial of some sort.

Therefore, when the time was right, Cait and I agreed to go and look for something by way of a memorial. We left it until the rawness had subsided then visited a stonemason on the outskirts of the city. Looking at shapes and sizes, wording and pictures, along with the various colours, we started to become overwhelmed with choices of gravestones. We had an idea of the wording we preferred. His grandmother had given us money to include the word *grandson* on the stone and we would also have *son* and *brother.* Checking out examples, there were also choices of having a picture of the deceased or items from their hobbies or interests carved into the stone. The saleswoman asked us a bit about Paul, we could only say he had been in the army. When she suggested a carving of a gun, I don't know how we kept our faces straight. A gun!

'We'll think about that,' was my reply.

We closed our gaping mouths, bit our lips and left before we burst out laughing. That was one of the days when we realised our keen sense of humour was returning. He now has his memorial, a stone with a simple message that will be there forever and this recollection is another memorial to my Little One.

And so, with the keys to his flat handed back, his will dealt with and his ashes handed over to us, it was time for the gravestone to be erected. Paul had died in his sleep on 2nd April but, because we didn't find him until four days later, the doctor was only able to provide a death certificate which read 6th April. This was the official date of his death and subsequently, the date which the stonemasons carved on his gravestone.

He's somewhere saying, 'You see, Mum, I told you… the system always gets it wrong! But who cares?'

THE END

www.ingramcontent.com/pod-product-compliance
Lightning Source LLC
Chambersburg PA
CBHW071156070526
44584CB00019B/2811